Casanova

How to Effortlessly Start Conversations and Flirt Like a Pro

Dave Perrotta

Copyright © 2021 Postgradcasanova

All rights reserved. No part of this book may be reproduced in any form without permission in writing from the author. Reviewers may quote brief passages in reviews.

Buyer Bonus

As a way of saying thank you for your purchase, I'm offering a FREE download that's exclusive to my book and blog readers.

It's a Texting "Cheat Sheet" that contains 18 powerful texts to capture her attention, get her on a date, and turn her on.

Inside you will learn:

-3 proven texts for setting up the date
-3 texts that turn her on and make her think about you
-A proven text that gets her to respond every time (even if she's been ignoring you)
-Simple online dating text openers for Tinder, OkCupid, etc. ...and much, much more.

Download it here:
postgradcasanova.com/conversation-casanova-free-ebook/

Dedication

This book is dedicated to all of the women in my life – past and present. You're all beautiful, intelligent, amazing, and you taught me more about myself than you can possibly know. You put up with my awkward jokes, my bad stories, and all the other BS.

Through the lessons you've directly (and indirectly) taught me, my life and my conversations will never be the same. It's also dedicated to my friends and family members who supported me while I researched and wrote the book. David, Danny, George, June, Mom, Dad – thank you all. I'm grateful for your support.

How to Tease Her the Right Way 96
Flirting Without Your Words 104
Part IV: Connect 109
Get Her Talking 110
How to Get Past Small Talk and Connect With Her 111
5 Go-To Conversation Topics for Connecting ... 126
Part V: Captivate 133
How to Talk About Yourself in an Attractive Way 134
How to Tell a Kick-Ass Story That Hooks Her In 154
Part VI: The Final Conversation 167
A Simple Habit to Improve Your Conversation Skills 168
How to Genuinely Love Women 172
The Final Talk 177
Bonus Chapter: 20 Questions to Ask a Girl on the First Date 179
Your Next Step 182
About the Author 183
How to Reach Me 185
A Parting Gift 186
Bonus Epilogue 187

Contents

Prologue: Straight Talk 7

"How Does He Make It Look So Easy?" 8

How to Use This Book 11

Who Am I to Write a Book About Conversation? 13

How to Master Conversation 19

Part I: The Casanova Mindsets (The Deeper Level of Conversation) 21

Why Your Mindsets are Crucial 22

Taking Responsibility for Your Life 25

Overcoming the Need for Validation 31

A Man With Purpose 35

"She's Into Me" 38

Part II: Initiate the Conversation 42

What to Do When You're Afraid to Approach Her 43

5 Ways to Start a Conversation With Any Girl 52

How to Make a Great First Impression 60

What to Say After You Start the Conversation 71

Part III: The Guide to Sexy Flirting 80

What is Flirting – And Why Do Most Men Suck at It? ....

The Biggest Key to Effective Flirting ....

Subtlety, Exaggeration, and Becoming the Prize

Prologue: Straight Talk

"How Does He Make It Look So Easy?"

"What the hell is he saying to her? How does he make it look so easy?"

You're out at the bar, and you see a normal-looking dude approach a beautiful girl.

Within minutes, she's completely enraptured by the conversation. Laughing, smiling, touching the guy – the whole nine yards. All the while, you sit back and wonder what type of magic spell this guy has put her under (and why you didn't go up and talk to her first!).

"Is he rich? Were they friends beforehand? Are they dating?" your brain starts to rationalize what's happening.

Before you know it, she has her phone out and she's giving him her number... or worse, she's leaving the bar with him! You're hit with feelings of jealousy and envy. You think back to your conversations where you couldn't "find the right word," or just couldn't "click" with the girl.

Has this ever happened to you?

It used to happen to me all the time. So, what are these guys saying? How are they connecting so quickly, flirting so easily, and attracting women so effortlessly?

Well, what you'll discover is that it's not all that complicated after all. The guys who "get it" – they all do similar things in conversation. They know how to make things sexual, make women laugh, have a good time, and connect with women.

What's more, you'll also discover a system so that you can easily replicate these types of conversations – and add in your own style. Sounds great, right? Hold on a second though...

You may be thinking, "What about all those studies that say '95% of communication is non-verbal'? Is conversation really that important?"

Fair point. But tell me, if you try and watch a movie in a different language (without subtitles), will you understand 95% of it?

Certainly not...

(Trust me, I've tried...)

Sure, there are a lot of things you can and should communicate non-verbally... But in order to truly connect with a woman, you need to use your words. This is how you find out her deeper aspirations, her personality, and whether or not she's the type of girl for you. This is how you ask her the questions that will give the interaction a deeper meaning.

What's more, this is how you make her FEEL something. And if you can make a woman feel good emotions, she can't help but be attracted to you.

Plus, the more you can connect with people through conversation, the more your world will open up to you.

Soon, you won't have to wonder how those guys make it "look so easy." Because YOU'LL be the guy who the other guys look at with jealousy, as you effortlessly attract women with your words.

Your dating life will be abundant, your relationships will flourish, and you'll have more opportunities than you can imagine.

So, how do you master conversation, connect with women, and harness the power of your words? Look no further than this book in your hands right now. It's a system that anyone can use to unlock the power of conversation.

Whether you're talking to women during the day, at the bar, or at your job – it doesn't matter. This conversation system will work anywhere.

So sit down and buckle up. The way you talk to people is about to change forever...

How to Use This Book

Anyone can pick up this book and read it – but not everyone will see results.

The difference between a man who uses this book to transform his conversation skills and the man who reads this book but fails to make changes is one small thing: *action*.

To get the most out of this book, you must do 2 things:

1. Be open to accepting new ideas.

2. Take action and implement the conversation strategies into your life.

When it comes to the dating realm, many men are closed off to new ideas. They think, "This is instinct. I already get it. I may not be having success with women right now, but it'll come. It's just a matter of time."

I get it man. Dating is a sensitive subject. Most men identify strongly with their ability to attract and date women (I know I did). And by opening themselves up to new ideas, they essentially question that ability. It's a tough blow to the ego.

But let me ask you a question...

How well have those ideas served you up to this point? If you're not having the success with women you want, and you're not connecting with women through conversations, then your ideas are holding you back.

In this book you'll learn a whole new approach to conversation and dating. I encourage you to read it with an open mind. You may be familiar with some of the concepts. You may have an urge to get defensive when I discuss the conversation "pitfalls." Instead of brushing them off and saying, "I would never make those mistakes," I encourage you to get introspective and be honest with yourself.

But you can't just read a book and expect it to get you results. Your results are dependent on the amount of action you take based on your reading. That's why I've made the system highly actionable. So, you can put it into use as you're reading.

If you do this, I can promise you your conversations will transform, you'll attract more women, and you'll start becoming the man you've always known you could be

But before we get into the system, I want to take a second to introduce myself, present my qualifications for writing this book, and tell you why I'm writing it...

Who Am I to Write a Book About Conversation?

You might be thinking, "Who is this guy, and what does he know about dating and conversation?"

I get it man. You've been fed shitty dating advice and creepy "pickup" tactics for years. You're not about to trust your dating life with a random schmuck.

So let me introduce myself. My name is Dave Perrotta. I'm a dating coach and the founder of PostGradCasanova. And while I can rant about how I've written multiple best-selling books, amassed over 55k subscribers on Youtube, and helped hundreds of thousands of guys improve their dating lives, I don't want to be a douche.

But I haven't always been good at talking to women and connecting through conversations. Things used to be A LOT different...

***

"David, you're going to be late!" my mom called out from down the stairs... I didn't care. I wanted to be late. I hated taking the bus to Hugh B. Bain

Middle School, back in my hometown of Cranston, Rhode Island because it always showed up to school early. Too early.

We'd have to stand outside for at least 15 minutes before the school doors opened. And for me, those 15 minutes felt like hours. All the other kids talked and socialized with each other. But I'd stand by the front stairs, alone, painfully searching for a group of acquaintances to "tag along" with.

I hated feeling like an outcast almost as much as I was afraid of conversing with new people. And yet, every morning for three years, I faced this uncomfortable fate. Thoughts like, "Am I really this much of a loser?" "Why can't I just talk to people?" "What do I say?" raced through my head…

I wanted to talk to people, but I was afraid they wouldn't accept me. I was afraid I wouldn't know what to say, and I'd be exposed as a loser. Everything in life seemed closed off.

You see, I was the "shy guy" in school. I grew up with a stutter, and the doctors thought I had Asperger's (a form of autism) until I was about 14 years old. Women felt like a different species, and the idea of conversation scared the hell out of me. I just wanted to hang in my room, avoid the world, and play video games.

Until one day, I couldn't do it anymore. I needed some sort of release. I needed to be a part of the world. I needed to have a fucking life. I wanted to date beautiful women. I wanted to connect with people. I wanted to be somebody. And I knew I couldn't do any of those things while I was locked up in my room. And so, my journey began.

It started off slow. As I tried to break out of my shell, I fell into common social traps, like trying too hard to fit in. I swore a lot because I thought it was cool, and I constantly got kicked out of class. I talked shit to people and got into fights (that I usually lost). I tried to flirt with girls, but failed miserably.

As the years passed and I grew, I started to make noticeable progress. Through trial and error, I started to learn how to connect with people. As I got more comfortable in my own skin, I learned how to flirt with women and become a bit funnier. At one point, I even had a girlfriend But by the time I started college, I still wasn't where I wanted to be.

So I made it even more of a point to improve. I read books, listened to programs, and took action – especially in the dating realm. I made more embarrassing mistakes with women than all my friends combined – but also talked to more people – and a lot more women – than all my friends combined. This was a huge part of my development, but it still wasn't enough.

So, once I hit 21 years old, I tried something new...

How I Finally Mastered Conversation After Years of Shyness and Rejection

It seemed clear what the missing piece was – I needed to be around guys who were good at talking to women. I needed to see what they were doing and how they were doing it. That way, I could figure out what I was doing wrong, and accelerate my progress.

So I asked myself, "How can I find guys who know this stuff?" After a quick Google search, I found a community in Boston of guys who went out and talked to girls.

Hesitantly, I signed up. A couple weeks later, I drove up to Boston and went to a group meetup. I had no idea what to expect. (Little did I know, this one night would completely change the trajectory of my life. It would be the start of a mental shift that would lead me to a life of entrepreneurship, world travel, and adventures I didn't even think were possible. What's even crazier is I would become great friends with 8-9 of these guys, and meet up with them all around the world [business conferences in Bangkok, parties in Colombia, etc.]. But that's a story for another time.)

We hit the club, and I quickly realized: many of these guys were "naturally" good at talking to women. All of their interactions seemed to flow smoothly. I knew I could learn a ton from these guys.

For the rest of that summer, I went out every weekend and watched closely as these "natural guys" seemed to attract women effortlessly. I saw the way they struck up conversations smoothly, made moves, and brought girl after girl back to their place...
I tried to mirror what they did, and I started getting better and better. But it was a slow process. I'd have some great conversations with women, yet sometimes, I'd fall flat on my face. Still, I constantly took action, interacted with women, and continued to learn.

I had some hiccups along the way – but as I learned from my mistakes, I made more progress. I was dedicated to the cause. Soon enough, I was going on 2-3 dates a week and sleeping with a new girl almost every weekend (all while I was broke and living with my parents)...

What I learned is you don't need to be rich, great looking, or have a great job to meet and attract women... But you DO need the right mindset, the confidence to approach and start conversations, and the ability to communicate sexually.

I also discovered that:

- You can learn how to get to know people on a deeper level

- You can learn how to be witty and make women laugh
- You can learn how to communicate sexually and turn women on
- You can learn how to give a woman the most amazing conversation she's ever had…every time.
- You can learn how to use conversation to get women irresistibly attracted to you and thinking about going home with you…minutes after first meeting you.

All of these things started happening to me as I mastered conversation. Armed with this knowledge and know-how, I started surpassing even the "natural" guys. That's when I realized, "I need to start helping other guys do this too…"

That was around 4 years ago. Since then, I've started PostGradCasanova where I've helped thousands of men improve their confidence, master conversation skills, meet more women, and have amazing sex lives. And now, I've distilled everything I've learned into one system that any man can use to master conversation and connect with women.

Whether you're broke, living with your parents, shy, or have been called "creepy" in the past… it doesn't matter. This system will give you the foundation and tools you need to be the kind of man who attracts any women he wants, connects with people, is the master of social situations, and has a thriving sex life.

How to Master Conversation

This book is divided into 6 key parts:

1. The Casanova mindsets (mastering the 4 mindsets that are essential to flirting with women)

2. Initiate the conversation (how to approach a girl and get the conversation going)

3. Flirt like a Casanova (communicate sexually and turn her on with your words)

4. Connect (how to develop the conversation and connect with women

5. Captivate (compel and attract women through conversation)

6. The final conversation (extra tips for making every conversation go well)

Part 1 will give you the mindsets of a man who attracts women through conversation. This will be your foundation.

Part 2 will help you start the conversation the right way, so you can develop it into something more.

Part 3 will give you the essentials for flirting and sexual communication. You'll learn how to make conversations more sexual, flirt, and turn women on with your words.

Part 4 will be your guide to connecting with women. You'll learn what to do and what NOT to do – so that your conversations flow smoothly and you can connect with women easily.

Part 5 will teach you to capture women's attention and attract them through conversation. You'll learn how to hook her in with stories and how to talk about yourself in an attractive way.

And finally, part 6 will give the remaining conversation strategies and tips you need to get through any conversation successfully. Now, it's time to dive into part 1: the deeper level of conversation. So roll your sleeves up and get ready!

Part I: The Casanova Mindsets (The Deeper Level of Conversation)

"Once your mindset changes, everything on the outside will change along with it." -Steve Maraboli

Why Your Mindsets are Crucial

Think of your mindsets as your foundation.

With a solid foundation, you can build something amazing and strong.

But with a shaky foundation, you have a house of cards. If one little thing goes wrong, it can send the whole thing toppling down – and you along with it.

Adding to that, a good mindset will help you to take the right action most of the time. Even if you've never faced a particular situation before, you'll be able to react calmly and efficiently…

On the opposite end, a negative mindset may cause you to freak out and react in an unhelpful way.

Your mindset is especially important when it comes to dating and conversation.

For example, let's say you've hung out with a girl a few times. Things seem to be going well – you have fun together and you seem to connect with each other easily.

But let's say you've unconsciously adopted a negative mindset, like "I need women to prove my self-worth."

So, when she doesn't text you back for a day, your mind starts flooding with insecurity. "Has she figured me out? I knew I wasn't good enough after all! Wait, who does this girl think she is? I'm gonna show her!"

Then, you lash out and tell her you deserve better and you can't believe she's being so inconsiderate.

She explains that she was just studying for a test, and she can't believe you're such an asshole. That's the last you hear from her.

You see, if you have a bad mindset, it doesn't matter how successful you are with women. The second you get a negative signal from a girl, it can trigger a downward spiral. That's because your confidence and self-worth will be dependent on the approval of women.

But with a good mindset, you can brush things off more easily and move on. What's more, you're far more likely to say the right things in conversation.

For example, if you have a positive mindset like, "All women are attracted to me until proven otherwise," you'll talk to a woman like she's attracted to you. In doing so, you'll be more flirtatious, confident, and naturally more sexual. You're far more likely to move the conversation towards what you want (like sex or a future date). Remember: Your mindsets dictate your thoughts, your thoughts dictate your actions, and your actions dictate your results.

Part I is all about diving into the 4 "Casanova mindsets" for flirting and conversation. Once you internalize these mindsets, everything else will become much easier.

So, follow along closely, do the action steps, and get ready for a mental shift.

Taking Responsibility for Your Life

The average guy won't have the success with women that he craves.

He will do okay (after all, there are a few billion women out there)…

But odds are, his dating trajectory will look something like this…

- He'll meet a few girls through his friends and college classes. He'll date a few here and there.
- When he graduates, he'll meet a girl or two from his work.
- Occasionally he'll go out, get drunk, and "get lucky" with a new girl at the bar or club.
- He'll get tired of the "single life" and start dating a girl from his social circle. The relationship will go on a little longer than it probably should.
- This cycle will continue until he eventually settles with a girl who he thinks is the "best he can do", though she doesn't really match up with his values or the traits he desires.
- He'll bicker to his friends about how his wife is always trying to "control him" and "take his freedom" and this will go on and on…
- Divorce, death, taxes, etc.

In short, he doesn't have much control over his dating life, or his life in general. It's highly dependent on the girls who sort of "stumble" into his life through work, friends, and drunken escapades.

But here's the thing: if you don't take control of your life, it's impossible to get what you want. Your results will be random. And you will not be happy with that randomness.

Here's an example...

I was an accounting major in college. A little more than half way through getting my degree, I started to have doubts about my career decision. "Do I really want to become an accountant? This whole thing seems a little...boring," I thought.

Although I had doubts, I also felt trapped. I'd already finished 2.5 years of school, and there was A LOT of pressure on me to continue. What else was I supposed to do? Switch my major? Drop out of school? And what would I tell my parents? Accounting was a secure career option. It was too hard to pass up.

"I'll just keep going with it for now and see what happens," I concluded. In doing so, I avoided taking control and responsibility of my life at that moment. I left my success and happiness up to mere chance. The result? I ended up suffering through the rest of my accounting classes and getting an accounting degree, followed by an office job that I hated.

Now, let's fast-forward a few years and see how things changed...

This time, instead of leaving things up to mere chance, I was fed up and determined to lead my life in the direction I wanted. I decided, "Enough is enough," and quit my accounting job. What I really wanted was the freedom to make money online, travel the world, and do work I was proud of.

So, I buckled down and started learning the necessary skills. After a few months, I was earning enough monthly income to move to Vietnam, where I knew there were hundreds of online entrepreneurs I could network with. So, I pulled the trigger and made the drastic life-change of moving to Asia.

In the two years since, I've lived in five different countries. I currently live on the beaches in Playa Del Carmen, Mexico, where I've learned Spanish, flirt with beautiful Mexican women, and love life. After this, I plan to keep traveling for years. It's the exact lifestyle I dreamed of a few years ago.

And the only reason it's possible is because I decided to take responsibility for my life.

You see, we don't always control what happens to us. But we always control a) how we interpret what happens to us, and b) how we respond to what happens to us. Therefore, whether we consciously recognize it or not, we are always responsible for our experiences and our life.

Casanova Mindset #1: I am responsible for my life and my circumstances.

Let's look at this through a dating lens again.

Think back to your failures with women (we've all had them)... There was always a reason for your failure. Sometimes you had control, and sometimes it was out of your control. But you have to remove the blame from women and take full responsibility.

For example:

- You're on a date with a girl, and the conversation is going well. You start telling her about your proudest accomplishments and hinting at how much money you make. She smiles and nods, but doesn't text you back after the date. **Why would she want a man who feels the need to constantly impress her? She can sense the insecurity.**

- You're sleeping with a girl and you start to become infatuated with her. You think about her all the time, and heap affection on her whenever you can. She seems happy at first, but quickly becomes more and more distant. Eventually, she backs off and asks for some time apart. Why would she want a man who makes a woman his main purpose?

These are situations where you'd be tempted to become bitter towards women. But instead, you need to manage your emotions, shift your perspective, and accept responsibility.

By taking responsibility, you can focus on what you need to improve, instead of getting bitter. Think of how this mindset will affect your conversations. With it, you'll understand that:

- It's your responsibility to make something happen with the girl

- It's your responsibility to lead the conversation in a positive way

- And you're responsible for the outcome of the interaction

In doing so, you will shift the way you look at conversation. And you'll be far more likely to take action on the nitty-gritty conversation tactics we'll talk about in Part II and beyond...

Also, think about how this mindset can affect your life...

You see, most people live reactive lives. They are slaves to their circumstances, and they react to whatever life throws at them. But in order to be successful in any area, you must take success into your own hands.

Realize that you have much more control over your circumstances and your life than you might think.

Action tip: Write down 2 things in your life that you feel like you're not taking full responsibility for. Then, write down how you can take control of these things right now...

For example, "I've put on some weight because I haven't been going to the gym. I can take control of this by finding a gym routine and sticking to it 3x a week."

Overcoming the Need for Validation

Deep down, most men believe they are inherently not "enough." They need other things to complete them, whether it be women, money, fame, etc. (or some combination of those).

They want to be respected by other men, and desired by attractive women.

This leads to needy behavior, because they're always trying to find the "missing piece."

This makes their conversations shallow, because they're always trying to "get something" out of the other person.

Here's the thing: You will never find that missing piece. There will always be more to desire.

Once you score a date with the girl, you'll want to bring her back to your place. Once you bring her to your place, you'll want to sleep with her. Then, you'll want to tell your friends about it and "show her off." That will be nice and feel good, but the good feeling will wear off.

Soon, you'll want more. You'll want to experience this feeling of approval again, and you'll need other women to fill the need. You'll need to keep trying harder to impress your friends and your parents. The cycle will never end.

If you're thinking, "I don't have this problem!" then I have a question for you...

Think of dating/picking up your dream girl. What excites you more? Experiencing her beauty, personality, and passion? Or bragging to your friends about getting such a 'hottie'?

Be honest with yourself.

For a long time, it was the latter for me. I approached and talked to women largely to impress other men. It was the only way I could prove my worth.

I remember back when I started college and pledged a fraternity. At that point, I had only slept with 1 girl. All the other fraternity guys bragged about sleeping with 10 or more. I felt like I wasn't enough – I needed more.

So I made it a point to sleep with as many women as possible – and brag about it as much as I could. I often came off shallow because women could tell I didn't care about them - I only wanted the validation they would give me. Now, I have a different perspective. When I see a girl, I don't think of the validation she can give me. Instead, I think, "She's attractive, and I want to talk her. I'll find out if she's cool, and if she is, maybe we can make something happen."

So, for you – how do you overcome the need for validation? That leads us to our second mindset...

Casanova Mindset #2: I am enough.

I don't need the approval of anyone else to feel complete. Many people live their life on "default mode." They don't take the time to analyze their true motivations and desires.

Often times, their motivations are based on getting approval from other people. For me, and maybe for you, this was the case.

 In doing so, they focus on living up to other people's values instead of their own. That's a recipe for failure.

Two of my biggest values are freedom and creativity. Back when I was studying accounting, I was living up to my parents' values of security and stability. This led to extreme unhappiness and stress.

But when I started focusing more on my values, I became much happier. Now, I enjoy the freedom I have to travel, as well as the creativity I can use to write books like this one.

When you focus on getting approval, you live up to other people's values. As you develop the mindset that "you are enough," you start living up to your own values.

Action tip: Write down your five most important values. Rate yourself from 1-10 on each value. For the categories you rate poorly, think of how you can improve and write it down.

For example, let's say you value freedom and wealth, but you're working at a time-consuming job that doesn't pay well. Maybe this means you start a "side hustle" so you can eventually quit your job, achieve more freedom, and make more money.

A Man With Purpose

We've all heard the quote, "If you don't know where you're going, any road will take you there."

Most men don't know where they're going. They're so focused on making a living that they forget to actually live.

This purposeless existence is terrible for building a life, and terrible for dating as well.

You see, women are attracted to men with purpose; a driving goal, propelling them forward despite the obstacles. Men with purpose don't depend on women's approval.

A man with purpose isn't affected by a bad conversation or two. Women know when they're talking to men with purpose because these men have a different look in their eyes. They know where they're going in a world where so many people are lost. They're striving for something, instead of "going with the flow" and blowing in the wind.

Mindset #3: Women are not my #1 priority. I have a mission and purpose outside of women.

You need to have a mission in life outside of women. Otherwise, you will be too tempted to give up on your passions and your direction in life and focus completely on women. Women will sense that they are the center of your world, and you won't be able to genuinely love them or connect with them. Instead, you will rely on them to fill needs that they cannot fill. This will undermine your conversations and your relationships.

Action Tip: Finding Your Purpose: Ask yourself, "What was a moment when I felt extremely energized and excited? And what was I doing at that time?" Write down your answer. By recognizing what makes you feel most alive and invigorated, you can better understand your motivations – this can help you clarify your purpose.

Thinking back to my early days, I always loved to write. I'd post multiple Myspace blogs every week. I also loved to be in front of large groups of people – I'd perform rap songs on chance every chance I could.

Through my blog, books, and videos, I have the privilege of doing both.

So dig deep with this action tip and ask yourself how you can start doing more of the things that make you come alive. By pursuing these passions, you'll give yourself the best chance to create a life you're truly proud of.

"She's Into Me"

Most women aren't going to come straight out and tell you they like you.

This poses a problem from most guys, especially if you're on the newer end of the spectrum.

You spend your time searching for signs that a woman is attracted to you (all while you don't really understand how to read those signs).

The result? You move slower with women as you struggle to read the signs. And when you don't get the signs you think you need, you avoid making a move. In doing so, you lose your chance with the girl.

But there is a solution to this...

You must assume attraction from all women until proven otherwise. And by "proven otherwise," I mean until she literally walks away or flat out tells you she isn't interested.

(Sidenote: Be smart about this. Obviously don't cross the line and make women uncomfortable with unwanted physical advances. If she says no, then stop.)

Mindset #4: All women are attracted to me until proven otherwise.

Is she dressed nice? It's because she's trying to impress you. She's playing with her hair? She's into you. She's standing with good posture? It's because she want you to notice her breasts and her butt popping out.

Every single sign she gives you is a sign of attraction and interest.

Compare this to the "innocent until proven guilty" nice guy approach. This guy writes off all those signs. For example: "Oh, she's playing with her hair? She must just be adjusting it;" "She made eye contact with me? Oh well, she probably has a boyfriend."

You must take the first approach. When you see and interact with women you're interested in, you must treat them like you're going to date them and bring them home.

This will change the way you talk to women, and also allow you to meet more women.

Think of all the ways this mindset can come in handy…

- You see a pretty girl sitting in the café? Assume she will be attracted to you and go introduce yourself.

- A cute girl from your improv class starts talking to you after class? Assume she's interested and ask if she wants to grab a drink.

- A girl is out with you on a date? Assume she wants to go home with you and ask if she wants to go back to your place for a drink.

- Texting a girl to try and get a date? Assume she's already interested and cut to the chase.

By assuming attraction, you'll give yourself the best chance with women in every interaction.

Assuming attraction won't make women magically fall all over you. If a girl isn't interested in you, "assuming attraction" won't be enough to flip her.

But if you approach them confidently, most women will be at least a little intrigued and open to you. By assuming attraction, you'll filter out the women who wouldn't have been into you anyway, and give yourself a much better chance of attracting the women who are at least open to you.

What's crazy is your reality starts to reflect your beliefs. When you assume women are attracted to you, you'll start acting like it. You'll make more sexual innuendos, lead women, and put yourself in a position to succeed. You'll be more comfortable interacting with women because you won't be worried about picking up on their signs of attraction.

Action Tip 1: Write down 2 thoughts that come to your head when you see a girl you're attracted to. Ask yourself: Are they empowering?

Action Tip 2: When you see a girl, imagine her responding very positively towards you. Then say to yourself, "This girl wants me"

This mindset will help you approach and lead women, make the move, and improve pretty much every other aspect of your dating life. It will also give you a big shot of confidence.

Part II: Initiate the Conversation

What to Do When You're Afraid to Approach Her

Before you can engage in a conversation, you must be able to start one.

Luckily for you, there are billions of women on the planet. So, it's not difficult to find one to start a conversation with.

And yet, so many men have trouble with this.

Why? Well, it's a combination of fear and insecurity.

They're afraid that women will reject them – and, even if they somehow make it through the first part of the conversation, they're afraid that they'll run out of things to say.

And so, they rarely initiate conversations. As a result, they don't meet nearly as many women as they should be meeting.

In the coming sections, you'll learn exactly what to say to keep the conversation flowing. But first, we have to get you through the beginning.

So let's tackle that fear of approaching…

***

You're in line at the supermarket. You look over to the next register line, and a beautiful girl catches your eye.

You admire her hair and her style, and you smile for a moment – she's exactly your type.

"Credit or debit?" the cashier repeats, as you snap back to reality and hand her your card. You sign the receipt and grab your bags – but when you look back to see the girl, she's gone.

"Damn!" you think to yourself. You missed your shot. But as you walk out the door, you see the same girl walking right in front of you.

You clam up for a second, wondering if you should make your move or let her go...

The excuses start flooding your brain... "She probably has a boyfriend..."; "She's a little too tall for me anyway..."; "She looks like she's in a rush..."; "I'd have to catch up to her to say 'hi' and that feels weird..."

What do you do next?

There are three possible scenarios:

1. You listen to your excuses, do nothing, and let her go.

2. You approach her and it goes well.

3. You approach her and it doesn't work out the way you wanted.

I was in this exact situation the other day. At first, I succumbed to my excuses – and I felt terrible about it.

But when she stopped on the street corner for a minute, I swallowed my pride and went for it.

The result? She gave me a big smile, and a minute or two later, I walked away with her phone number and plans for drinks later this week.

I felt the fear, and did it anyway.

So – what was going through my head then – and what can you do to propel yourself forward when you're afraid to approach her?

How can you start seizing the opportunities instead of letting them slip through your fingers?

It comes down to the following 4 actions...

1. Focus on Overcoming Your Fear

If you're afraid to approach her, it actually works in your favor.

You see, boldly confronting your fear can feel far more rewarding than simply starting a conversation with a random girl.

One of the greatest discoveries a man makes, one of his great surprises, is to find he can do what he was afraid he couldn't do. – Henry Ford

When you focus on confronting and overcoming the fear, you'll not only approach more women, but you'll also grow as a man.

You'll realize, "I had these excuses. I had this story I was telling myself. But I approached her anyway. I did what I was afraid I couldn't do." – and it will feel awesome.

2. Shift Your Perspective

Often the reason you're afraid to approach her is because you feel like it's too risky. She could reject you and damage your ego. Or maybe she'll respond well, but then you'll run out of things to talk about.

In the moment, these fears are perfectly reasonable. It's easier and more comfortable for you to do nothing than to take action. The risk of rejection and embarrassment doesn't feel worth it.

When you're afraid to approach her, your risk spectrum looks like this:

Risk of approaching her: You'll have an awkward interaction, get rejected, and feel terrible – a big risk.

Risk of doing nothing: No risk – you'll save your ego, stay in your comfort zone, and move on like nothing happened.

But you need to shift your perspective, so that it's actually more risky not to approach her.

You need to adjust your understanding of the risks, so that:

Risk of approaching her: Potential awkward interaction with a girl you'll probably never see again. So, 1-2 minutes of discomfort – a small risk.

Risk of doing nothing: You miss out on a potential amazing connection and incredible sex with a woman you're attracted to – a big risk.

Risk of building the habit of not approaching: You signal to your subconscious that it's "okay" not to approach women you're interested in. In doing so, you miss out on other great girls in the future – another big risk.

With this perspective, it's more risky for you to do nothing than to approach her.

Use this reversal of risk to propel you forward and get the women you want. Make a conscious effort to view approaching women from this perspective.

It is better by noble boldness to run the risk of being subject to half the evils we anticipate than to remain in cowardly listlessness for fear of what might happen. – Herodotus

3. Stop Waiting for the Right Moment

Don't waste time waiting for the right moment. You won't find it – you'll always have an excuse in your head as to why it's the wrong moment.

Instead of waiting, make a habit of taking a step in the direction of the girl you want to talk to. Don't comb your brain for the perfect thing to say, and don't pause.
Just start walking towards her.

She could be talking to her friend, on the phone, eating lunch at an outdoor patio – it doesn't matter. If you don't talk to her now, you probably won't get another chance – and if you wait too long, you'll build up the fear in your head and psyche yourself out.

As I always say, if you point out a girl and tell me to approach her now, I can do it – no problem. But if you point a girl out and tell me to approach her in 5 minutes? Well that's a whole different ballgame. It's going to be A LOT tougher because I'll be building it up in my head for those five minutes, as opposed to if I just took immediate action.

So, take the first step. The action will help you conquer the fear.

Listen to your excuses and let them go.

4. Tap Into Your Manhood

Why do you want to approach her? At some level, she gives you the feels. You find her sexy and intriguing.

But often, you leave your attraction on the backburner, and instead focus on the fear of approaching.

All of these thoughts start going through your head. "Does she like me?" "Should I try to kiss her?" "What should I talk about?" "What if she thinks I'm boring?"

Instead, you need to keep your attraction and appreciation for her beauty on the forefront of your mind. This will help you cultivate a nervous excitement instead of a nervous fear. An excitement to meet and learn more about her.

How do you do that?

Ask yourself: What do you like about her?

Do her eyes draw you in and captivate you? Is her smile contagious? Is her rhythm sexy? Does she make you laugh? Bring these thoughts to the forefront of your mind.

As you appreciate her inner and outer beauty, you'll be more in tune with your natural male instincts.

For me, it always brings a smile to my face and leads me to make strong eye contact. It allows me to be more free flowing and in the moment as well.

When you approach her with this excitement, often she will mirror you. Even if she isn't into you at first, she'll begin to find you intriguing and feel the same type of excitement.

So, tap into your manhood and focus on what you find attractive about her – this will make it easier to approach, and the girl will usually respond better.

***

Listen man. The fear of approaching a new girl will always be there. You can never completely eliminate it. But that's okay – you don't need to.

A little fear is what makes the process fun and rewarding.

So, keep these 4 actions in mind to help you conquer fear when you feel like it's overwhelming you.

To recap, here are the 4 actions for overcoming your fear of approaching her:

1. Focus on overcoming your fears

2. Shift your perspective

3. Stop waiting for the right moment

4. Tap into your manhood

Once you conquer your fear, you still need to know how to start the conversation. That's what we'll talk about next...

5 Ways to Start a Conversation With Any Girl

You now have 4 concrete actions to conquer your fear of approaching women. But once you approach them, what do you say? How do you start the conversation?

Well, what you say to start the conversation depends on a few things, like:

- **The environment.** The way you start a conversation during the day may be a bit different than the way you start the conversation at a nightclub.

- **The girl.** If she's in a rush, you'll have to move the conversation quickly. Whereas, if she's standing and watching a street performer, you know she has some time, and there are plenty of things to talk about.

- **Your goals.** Maybe you're not super interested in the girl and you just want to build some social momentum. Or, maybe your intuition literally forced you to talk to this girl because she caught your eye so strongly.

Whatever the situation, this chapter will help you start the conversation well and move things forward with the girl.

(Keep in mind – when you're in a naturally social environment, like perhaps a social sport, house party, or a get together with new friends, you can be pretty casual with the way you start a conversation. That's because it's expected to be social in these types of situations. We'll go over this as well.)

We'll talk about 5 easy ways you can start a conversation with any girl…

Let's get right into it…

1. Going "Direct"

Here, you basically state your interest from the beginning. This is one of my favorite ways to start a conversation, because it cuts through the bullshit.

When it's best to use: Anytime.

You can say:

"Hey, I know this is really random, but I saw you walking by and I thought you were cute. So, I had to say 'Hi'. I'm [Your name]."

It's very important to say this one slowly and shake her hand afterward. You want to say it like this...

"Hey... I know this is reaaaallly random... but I saw you walking by... and I thought you were cute... So I had to say 'Hi'...I'm [Your name]."

By delivering it slowly, you'll come across as more confident and she'll hang on your words. By shaking her hand, you'll initiate physical touch from the beginning, which will make her more comfortable with you.

Going "direct" is powerful because it shows confidence, and if she stays in the conversation, it's a sign that she's at least somewhat interested in you.

2. Situational

Here, you pick out something from the environment, and use it to start the conversation.

When it's best to use: At a bar or club, or when the two of you are stationary (in one place, perhaps looking at something like a street performer).

For example, let's say the two of you are staring at one of those street performers who pose as a statue. You could say, "I always confuse these things with real statues. My friends always make fun of me for it." This is a fun, tongue-in-cheek way to initiate the conversation.

If you're in a bar or club, you could even say something simple like, "Do you know what the name of this club is?"

The key is to deliver this with a slight smile, so she knows you're being playful. You want it to come across in more of a fun way rather than a serious tone.

The "situational" conversation starter can be powerful because it already gives you a topic to discuss. It can also be a great way to make her laugh from the beginning. However, make sure not to stay on the topic too long, as it can go stale and get boring. There's only so much you can say about a street performer.

3. The "Where is Starbucks?"

You're walking down the street and you stop a girl, then ask her where the nearest Starbucks is.

When it's best to use: During the day while you're walking in a city that has Starbucks (if that city doesn't have Starbucks, any other popular café/restaurant will do).

Here's the key to pulling this one off...

First, spot the girl you want to talk to. Typically, she'll be walking towards you on the sidewalk.

Once you're within 10 feet of her, slowly raise your hand in front of you to get her attention. She'll usually see your hand and your eye contact before she gets to you.

Then, plant your feet and stop in front of her.

Ask, "Hey, do you know where the nearest Starbucks is?"

Before she can fully respond, cut her off and say, "Actually, I just thought you were cute and I wanted to meet you. I'm [Your name]."

(It's important to do this BEFORE she finishes giving you the directions, because the social tendency is to give the quick directions and immediately walk away.)

This conversation starter is powerful because it allows you to gauge her vibe and attractiveness before you show your interest. For example, simply by her response and the way she starts to deliver her answer, you can tell how open she is to having a conversation with you. For example, if she smiles and lights up little bit, you know you have a good chance to make something happen.

Plus, if she's not as attractive as you thought she was from afar, you can just ask the Starbucks question and let her give you the directions, then walk away. It's very low risk.

4. The Simple Introduction

Here, you don't try to get too cute. You just give her a simple, "Hey, how's it going? Or, "Hey, I'm [Your name]. How's it going?"

When it's best to use: At bars and clubs and other social environments.

It's important to deliver this with confidence, strong eye contact, and a lower tone of voice. Otherwise, you'll come across in a platonic "just friends" sort of way, and you'll often get brushed off by women.

It's powerful because of its simplicity. You don't have to dig for what to say. You know that you have this simple conversation starter in your back pocket.

5. The Seahorse vs Octopus

I'll go out on a limb here and say you probably haven't heard of this one… Typically I'm not a huge fan of routines and opinion type of conversation starters. When my friend came to me with this conversation starter, I laughed out loud. Then, I saw him use it over and over again – and women would light up (he'd often bring them home).

I started using it as well – and it got me some hilarious (and very satisfying) results.

When it's best to use: Anytime, but especially at night in bars and lounge types of places.

Here's how to use it...

You go up to a group of girls and say, "My friends and I have been having an interesting discussion and wanted your input."

Once they oblige, you say, "I'm thinking of getting a more non-traditional pet. And it's between a seahorse and an octopus. Which would you get?"

What I've found is that girls typically have a weird obsession with one of those two animals – and they light up when you ask the question.

It's powerful because it's a very fun way to start the conversation, and engages women right away. Plus, it's great to use when you're talking to groups of women.

***

There you have it – you now have 5 ways to start a conversation with any women and in any environment. You no longer have an excuse to not approach and start conversations with women you desire.

Now, it's time to put this knowledge into action.

Action Tip: Pick at least one of these conversation starters and use it THIS week. Feel free to send me an email with how you do at Dave@PostgradCasanova.com!

As you read through this book and take action, you're going to get better at every step of conversation. You'll improve your delivery of these conversation starters so that you get better responses, and you'll also become more comfortable with starting conversations.

But for now, do the action tip! And get ready to learn a whole lot more...

How to Make a Great First Impression

It's important to start the conversation – but what's perhaps even more important is the first impression you give off.

You can have the smoothest line in the world – but if you're not saying it the right way or you're making awkward movements, it won't matter. Women will shut you down and you'll be back to the drawing board.

The way you say your words and move your body is just as important as the actual words themselves.

They all come together to form your first impression.

So, how do you make a great first impression? You must 1) avoid common mistakes and 2) speak and move your body in the right way.

In this chapter, we'll go over common first impression mistakes, help you correct them, and get you making great first impressions in no time.

Let's get started.

First Impression Mistake #1: Talking Too Fast

"If I don't get out my words quickly enough, she'll stop paying attention or walk away..."

Thoughts like these sweep through our subconscious mind as we speed up our words.

But put yourself in a girl's shoes for a second.

A guy approaches you and speeds through his introduction so quickly, you barely understand a word he says. Then, when you ask him to repeat himself, he speeds through it again.

How would this make you feel? Probably pretty uncomfortable, right?

Solution #1: Slow It Down

The slower you talk, the more you will captivate women. The faster you talk, the more you signal that you're insecure.

As a rule of thumb, slower is better. But when you're a little nervous and talking to a girl, you can lose track of this. You start talking faster because it's a nervous habit. This makes her uncomfortable and kills the vibe.

Instead of a slow, controlled introduction, like:

"Hey…I know this is random… but I just saw you walking by… and you caught my eye…and I wanted to say hi… I'm Dave…"

It turns into:

"HeyIKnowThisIsRandomButIsawyouwalkingbyando mgIhadtosayhiImdaveHowareyoudoingwhatareyouu ptoomgyourehotahhh."

Not exactly the best way to start the conversation…

So, work on slowing down your speech. Be aware of the speed that you talk, and slow it down to the point where it feels like it's too slow. Then, slow it down another notch from there. That's usually the right speed for creating a good vibe.

This alone has changed the game for many of my dating coaching clients. It's helped them to connect with women and have far better conversations. If you remember nothing else from this book, remember this point and slow things down.

First Impression Mistake #2: Speedy, Anxious Movements

Picture an unconfident man walk into a club. How does he look?

He probably makes uncomfortable, jittery movements. He jerks his head around, as he scans the club rapidly. And when he walks around, it doesn't seem like he has any sort of purpose.

Instead, he walks fast and seems lost – even intimidated.

Have you ever seen the movie Limitless? Well, you could compare this guy to the main character of that movie when he's not on the brain-enhancing drug.

This man is clearly not comfortable with his surroundings. Now, perhaps you say, "I'd never be like that guy!"

But chances are, you've had your moments where you make jittery movements. And chances are, you occasionally fidget around when you're talking to girls.

Perhaps you peel the wrapper off a beer can, shake your leg, or touch your face. Whatever it is, you better believe women notice.

Solution #2: Slow Down Your Movements

Powerful and attractive men move slower.

Where an insecure man might walk fast and slouch with his head down, an attractive man will walk slowly down the street with his back straight, smiling at the women who pass by.

When you slow your movements down, you'll come off as more confident and appealing.

This is especially important in a bar/club setting. Simply walking slowly and smiling will make women notice you, and they'll start giving you approach invitations (AKA signs that they want you to approach them, like making eye contact with you, playing with their hair, etc.).

And when you approach them, the interaction will instantly have a sexual undertone.

In the past few years, I've witnessed this phenomenon first-hand. When I was younger, women would hardly ever toss me looks of interest. But now, whether I'm walking through the club or even on the sidewalk, I constantly get "gazes of interest" from women. It makes things a lot easier.

First Impression Mistake #3: Looking Too Serious or Too Goofy

On one end of the spectrum, you have the guy who never smiles. Whenever he's in a conversation, he takes it seriously – too seriously.

The girl thinks, "Why does this guy seem like he has a stick up his ass the whole time?"

You never want to be the guy who takes himself too seriously...

Then on the other end of the spectrum, you have the goofy guy.

This guys smiles wider than the Kool Aid Man after bursting through a wall. This is the "friendly/goofy" smile that literally screams "just friends!"

(Think Erkle's smile after he says his famous line, "Did I do that?!")

You don't want to be the goofy smile guy either. Instead, you need to strike a balance.

Solution #3: The Sexy Smile

Smiling is crucial, especially because of the phenomenon of mirror neurons. Basically, these are brain cells that cause us to feel the same emotion as we see others feeling.
But you have to get your smile right. Don't be like Erkle. Instead, aim for the type of smile that Ryan Gosling constantly uses in the movie Crazy, Stupid, Love.

Here are the characteristics of a "sexy" smile:

- Show very little teeth (or just keep your mouth shut)

- Smile with one side of your mouth more than the other

- It's almost a "half smile" or slight grin, whereas the friendly guy's smile is very broad

This is something you want to get down pat, because many women will judge you based on your smile. If you're tired of being stuck in the friendzone, nail this one down.

First Impression Mistake #4: Slouching

Growing up, I naturally had bad posture. My back is curved, and when I'm sitting, I occasionally look like the hunchback of Notre Dame.

This is something I've had to deal with – and I've had to consciously adjust my posture.

Why? Because I know how damaging bad posture can be. When you slouch, it signals to women that you're insecure and unconfident.

Look around the room the next time you go out. You can usually tell the guys who get laid from the guys who don't, simply based on the way they move and position their bodies.

(Hint: the guys who have success with girls don't slouch and put their head down.)

Solution #4: Develop Strong Posture

Be aware of the way you move your body. Practice walking with your head high, shoulders back, and your body straight.

Yoga can also be extremely helpful. I started doing yoga twice a week, and after two months, I've already noticed a huge difference. I'm more flexible and comfortable in my body, and my posture has improved A LOT.

As a bonus, yoga is a great place to meet beautiful, fit women who are in tune with their bodies.

First Impression Mistake #5: Darting Eyes

Have you ever talked to someone who makes strong eye contact with you? It can be intense, and even a little intimidating at times.

Deep down, you know this person is confident and comfortable; otherwise they wouldn't be able to hold such strong eye contact.

On the other hand, have you ever talked to somebody with darting eyes? They're talking to you, but their eyes are floating around the room. They're looking up, down, and all around, but rarely into your eyes.

It almost seems like they're trying to hide something. It's a weird feeling.

Darting eyes like these will ruin a first impression.

Solution #5: Strong Eye Contact

Eye contact is powerful – the brain sends out relationship-building chemicals like oxytocin when you make eye contact with somebody.

One study from the Journal of Research in Personality found that simple eye contact could actually make a person fall in love with you. [1]

...But you need to be able to make eye contact without being creepy. When you talk to women, focus on holding it for around 70% of the time. Look at her right eye, so your eyes don't shift back and forth.

When you make eye contact from the other side of the bar/club or in general, hold it until she looks away. Then, once you've made eye contact, walk towards her and approach her.

Good eye contact is something you must learn – so the more you practice, the better.

First Impression Mistake #6: Talking With a High-Pitched Voice

Here's another tendency of nervous men: They talk with a higher-pitched voice.

This is an instant turn-off for women, and will get you labeled in the "just friend" category.

Chances are, you're speaking with a higher pitch than you should be. That's because when you're nervous, you tend to speak from your throat.

This causes you to come across in a platonic, nonsexual way. It ruins the potential for a sexual connection.

Solution #6: Speak from Your Belly

Practice speaking from your belly and projecting your voice.

To do this, focus on maintaining a deep breathing pattern. Breathe in through your nose, and deep into your belly. You should feel your stomach rise and fall with each breath.

Practice this in private – that way, it feels more natural when you're with a girl.

We tend to speak where we breathe from. If you breathe from your throat, you'll probably have a weak, high-pitched voice. But if you speak from your belly, your voice will likely be deeper and more masculine, which is essential for a good first impression.

***

By avoiding these mistakes and taking the right actions, you'll immediately improve your first impressions. This will allow you to connect with women and sexualize the conversation much easier.

However, you still need to know what to say after you've started the conversation and made a good first impression. That's what the next chapter is all about.

Reference:

1. Kellerman, Joan, James Lewis, and James D. Laird. "Looking and loving: The effects of mutual gaze on feelings of romantic love." Journal of Research in Personality 23.2 (1989): 145-161.

What to Say After You Start the Conversation

"Hey, I know this is random, but I saw you walking by and you caught my eye. I had to meet you. I'm [Your name]," you say.

"Wow, thanks! I'm Jessica," she replies and shakes your outreached hand.

The conversation shifts back to you. At that precise moment, your mind goes blank.

You mutter something bland, like "Yeah it's good to meet you…" without adding any more value to the conversation.

"Yes, it is! But I have to run! Have a good day!" she says.

And just like that, in a split second, you miss your opportunity.

Sucks, right?

We've all been in that type of situation before. We start off well, but then go blank, and the conversation stalls.

So, how can you prevent this? What should you say and do after you approach her?

That's what this chapter is all about.

Before you do anything else, you should introduce yourself. All you need to say is something simple like, "I'm Dave by the way."

She'll usually respond with her name, and when she does, you should shake her hand. This helps build an initial level of comfort, and makes it seem like the two of you aren't strangers anymore.

But where do you take it from there?

The First Question

Once you do the intro, there's a key question you should follow up with...

This question is so simple, you'll kick yourself for not thinking of it earlier.

Heck, you might even use it now, but you probably don't understand its power (and so you're using it wrong).

Here's the question: "What are you up to?" (I told you it was simple, right?) It's powerful because it can instantly tell you her logistics. You'll know:

- If she's in a rush

- If she has a few minutes to talk

- If she has a lot of time (As you'll see in a minute, this is very important information.)

You may get responses like:

- "I'm on my way back to work!"

- "I'm just hanging out and doing a little shopping."

- "I'm meeting a friend in a little while."

These responses will present you with 3 different types of situations – along with several directions for which you can take the conversation.

Let's look at these situations you'll face after approaching a girl for the first time – as well as how you can handle each.

Situation #1: She's in a Rush

She stops to talk to you, but she's clearly in a rush and has to do something. You can usually pick up on this through her vibe, or simply by the way she answers your "What are you up to?" question.

So, what should you do if you've only got a minute or less to talk to her?

A lot of guys think this isn't enough time to do anything, but they're wrong.

If you think she's attractive and you'd like to see her again, you should STILL ask for her number. It doesn't matter that you've just met her – you literally have nothing to lose.

Here's what you should say if she's in a rush:

"I know this is random and we literally just met, but you have a really fun/interesting vibe. We should grab a drink this week or next."

By saying "I know this is random and we just met," you signal that you have social intelligence (because you're aware of the randomness of the situation), while also addressing her potential objection of "But we just met!" BEFORE she can say it.

If she says, "Yeah, that sounds fun!" you can say, "Okay, awesome!"
Then pull out your phone, bring it to the "add contact" screen, hand it to her, and tell her to put her number into your phone.

If she says something along the lines of "No" followed by an excuse (like "I have a boyfriend"), you can say, "No worries, just take it as a compliment then," and leave the conversation.

Situation #2: She Has a Few Minutes to Talk

She lets you know she's meeting up with a friend in a few minutes, or perhaps at the beginning of her lunch break from work. You can tell she's not in a huge rush, but she does have somewhere to be in a little while.

Your goal here should be to make a good first impression, and get her number at a high point in the conversation. All you really have to do here is make an assumptive statement (i.e. make a guess about her).

There are three types of assumptive statements you can make:

1. Where she's from: "You look like you're from New York."

2. What she does for a living: "You seem like you do something creative."

3. What type of person she is: "You seem like a fun, adventurous kind of person."

These statements will give you some good, fun conversational material. From here, you should be able to keep the conversation going for 2-3 minutes.

Then, when the conversation seems to be at a high point (the two of you are laughing, realize you have something in common, etc.), tell her you need to go, and ask for her number.

You can say something like, "Listen, it's been great to meet you. I gotta go, but you seem like a lot of fun. We should grab a drink this week or next."

Once she says "Yes!" pull out your phone and have her put her number in.

Situation #3: She's Got a Lot of Time on Her Hands

After approaching her, you realize she's not really doing much right now. She's not in a rush and she doesn't have to be anywhere.

Here, you have two options:

1. Take her on an "instant date"

2. Talk to her for a little while and grab her number (similar to if she has a few minutes to talk)

We'll get to both of these scenarios in a second – but let's talk about some more conversational tools you can use to extend the conversation.

Aside from making statements, you can also:

- Ask open-ended questions (like, "What brings you to X city?"), then listen and relate back with your own experiences

- Compliment her in genuine and unique ways (like, "You have a very unique style. I might need to get some fashion tips from you")

- Playfully tease her (i.e. Oh you're from LA? You're a Valley girl at heart, aren't you?")

These tips will help you extend the conversation and connect with her.

(We're going to go over all of these conversational tactics throughout the rest of the book— this is just a brief introduction to them.)

Okay, now let's get back to those two options we mentioned before...

How to Take Her on an "Instant Date"

Here, you can say, "I'm not in a big rush right now and you seem like fun. I know a great ice cream/coffee place down the street. What do you say we check it out?"

The benefit of an "instant date" like this is that it can create a deeper connection and more familiarity with the girl. The danger is it can lead to you getting friendzoned.

For it to work well, you need to maintain the flirtatious, man-to-woman type of vibe throughout the interaction (which can sometimes be difficult in a daytime setting if you don't have a lot of experience).

As for the second scenario (talk to her for a little while and grab her number), you basically just do the same thing as you would if she had a few minutes to talk. Maybe you stay in for a few extra minutes and use the three conversation tips from this section. Then, you get her number at a high point in the interaction and leave.

You now have a solid structure to handle most of the situations when you'll be approaching a girl. Internalize this structure, and you won't have to worry about "running out of things to say" after you approach her. You'll be able to make the conversation interesting and connect with her.

In doing so, you'll give yourself the best chance to get her number and see her again.

Action Tip: Approach a girl today or tomorrow. Use one of the conversation starters from the last section, and follow it up by introducing yourself and asking, "What are you up to?"

Part III: The Guide to Sexy Flirting

What is Flirting — And Why Do Most Men Suck at It?

Flirting is the way you arouse a girl's interest and make her picture the two of you together romantically. It's essential to your conversations with women. Without it, you'll have platonic conversations and constantly get labeled as the "just a friend" guy.

There are two types of flirting: friendly flirting and sexual flirting. Friendly flirting is innocent. It's how most men communicate with the women they desire. With sexual flirting, there are sexual undertones. Girls won't mistake this type of flirting as "just friend" flirting. THIS is how you should aim to flirt with the women you desire.

Here are some examples:

- Breaking eye contact quickly (friendly) vs looking at her seductively (sexual)

- "What do you like most in a guy?" (friendly) vs "What do you find sexiest in a guy?" (sexual)

The unfortunate thing (or, perhaps fortunate for us guys who work on our flirting skills) is that most men suck at flirting.

Why? It comes down to 3 main reasons...

1) They're Too Blunt

Bluntness isn't exciting for women. The reason? When you're blunt, you leave no room for intrigue. The fun is gone. Here's an example:

Her: "I love lingerie."

You: "I bet you look amazing in lingerie."

As you'll see in the next chapter, great flirting is much more subtle. There's more mystery involved. More for the woman to guess about.

2) They're Too Forward

Being too forward also ruins the mystery.

Here's an example:

Her: "Yeah, at one point the French colonized Vietnam."
You: "Oh really? Well I'd like to colonize you..."

Aside from ruining the mystery, it can also trigger sexual shame in women. I remember one night in a Boston club 4 or 5 years ago. I had been partying with a sexy Asian girl, and we were hitting it off. The logistics were good, her friends were cool with it, and all signs pointed to us going home together.

Then, as we were in line at the coat check, I said something like, "I can't wait to get back... I'm going to f**k you so hard later." She seemed into it. But no more than 5 minutes later, she made an excuse as to why she could no longer go home with me. The mood had completely shifted.

Why? Because I was way too sexually forward. She could no longer tell herself, "I'm just going back with this guy to have fun, and we'll see what happens." Instead, she had to tell herself, "I'm going back to have sex with this guy." Sure, maybe she wanted sex at the time, but this was too much for her. She could no longer rationalize her decision, and by going home with me, she likely would have felt "wrong" or "dirty."

3) They Use Friendly Flirting Instead of Sexual Flirting

Friendly flirting is the easy route. It's innocent, and doesn't require much risk. If you try to "high five" a girl, she'll usually do it. But if you try to hold hands with her and play with her fingers? Well, that's much more bold and risky.

Most guys go with friendly flirting. As a result, they're interactions lack any sort of sexual undertone.

So, how can you avoid these mistakes and embrace the art of sexy flirtation? That's what this section is all about...

The Biggest Key to Effective Flirting

Flirting is an art that few men have mastered.

As you'll see throughout this section, there are several aspects of effective flirting. But before you start nailing down those aspects, you must first learn the most important element of flirting:

Intent.

*** "What were you doing, bro? What was that?"

My friend had just approached a girl here in Playa Del Carmen, Mexico. I was sitting beside him, so I heard the whole thing.

Him: "Where are you from?"

Her: "Merida!" Him: "Ah cool. I heard Merida was a cool city to visit."

Her: "Yeah it's a great city to live in and there's tons of tourist stuff too…"

Him: "Cool. What do you think of it compared to Playa Del Carmen?"

…

He was clearly attracted to her, but the conversation was painfully platonic. It wasn't so much what he was saying (he was attempting to flirt), but the way he was saying it.

Instead of sounding like a man who was sexually interested her, he sounded like a flimsy tourist.

MOST guys come across in this very platonic way when they approach or talk to girls.

Can you relate?

You see, this creates a weird dynamic with the girl. You approach her because you're interested, and you even say some of the right things, yet you communicate with her in a friendly, platonic way. It's not congruent, and it puts her in an awkward situation. *"Why is this guy even talking to me?"* she's thinking.

The conversation isn't sexually charged, because you're not speaking like a man and communicating with sexual intent.

But wait – why should you communicate with sexual intent?

- It destroys any chance of you being in the friendzone

- It communicates that you're a sexual guy who goes for what he wants

- It's the foundation of building sexual attraction

- Women will be a lot more likely to see you again

- It sexually charges your conversations

Put simply, in her mind, it's the difference between being intrigued (i.e. "Mmm, who is this guy?") and being slightly annoyed or bored (i.e. "Why is he talking to me? I need to leave...").

I took my friend aside to explain. "Look man, it doesn't matter what you're saying to her. It's the way you say it and the intent behind it. You need to communicate with intent.

Think for a second...Why do you even bother approaching girls in the first place?

In my friend's case, he approached the girl because he was attracted to her. And yet he communicated with her like a confused tourist. He spoke with no intent.

You usually approach a girl because you're attracted to her. There's something about her that you find sexy. But throughout your whole life, you've been programmed to cover up your sexual desires. You've basically been told to hide the fact that you're a man thanks to all the terrible advice and political correctness in the media.

But you are a man, so you should act like one. The girl should have no doubt that she's speaking to a sexual man who goes for what he wants.

Your intent should come through in all the words you say. Even if you ask, "Do you know where the nearest Starbucks is?" you should sub-communicate something like, "I think you're sexy and I want to know more."

On the surface, here's what it looks like to communicate with intent:

- Hold strong eye contact

- Talk slower

- Smile

Below the surface, you're thinking:

- I might want to hook up with this girl and I'm okay if she picks up on this vibe

- She is attracted to me

- I choose the women I want in my life

This takes some work – but once you can start communicating with intent, your conversations with women will transform.

Keep this in mind as we go through the rest of this section. Everything you'll learn here will help you to communicate with intent.

Sound good? Okay, now let's move on to the aspects of sexy flirting...

Action Tip: Communicate with at least 3 women with intent.

Subtlety, Exaggeration, and Becoming the Prize

This is a conversation I've had many times over the years...

Her: "How old are you?"

Me: "How old do you think I am?"

Her: "I don't know, 31, 32?"

Me: "I'm 50, but I work out a lot."

Her: "[Laughing] Get out of here! You're ridiculous. How old are you really?"

Me: "I'm 25. What about you?"

Her: "What?! 25? I'm 31!"

Me: "31? Wow, you're way too old for me. This would never work. You're just going to try to take advantage of me and all my innocence."

The conversation is a quick back and forth, with a lot of flirting involved. And a lot of times, that's what flirting is: it's quick, it's witty, and it's fun.

It's also the direct opposite of the mistakes we talked about in the first chapter of this section (being blunt, overly direct, and too friendly).

In this chapter, we'll talk about some of the conversational aspects of sexy flirting: subtlety, exaggeration, and positioning yourself as the prize.

These aspects will help you become a master at witty banter.

Using Subtlety

Think back to the example from a few chapters ago of being overly direct…

Her: "I love lingerie."

You: "I bet you look amazing in lingerie."

Now, let's look at a more subtle way you could do this…

Her: "I love lingerie."
You: "Really? Well I know it may sound crazy, but I love women who love lingerie."

Can you feel the difference in these two examples?

In both examples, you're saying that you like the girl. But the second is much more subtle.

Why? It's all about the implication.

There's a difference between explicitly saying that you like a girl (or that you want to have sex with her, kiss her, etc.) and implying it. The latter is much more exciting to women.

With the implication, there's more of a challenge. You show that you're interested in her, but you don't reveal all of your cards. It's enough to keep her around and engaged, but not so much that it ruins the moment.

Not only that, but it also shows that you have standards. You're not just blindly attracted to any girl with decent looks and a pretty smile.

Whereas when you're blunt and clumsy with your words, you seem more like a guy who's drooling over her than a high value guy she should be attracted to.

Subtlety and implication are key.

Exaggeration

If you're talking to a high-quality woman, she's usually going to try to test you at some point. These tests usually come in the form of verbal jabs. She wants to see how you respond. If you pass, she knows you're confident in yourself and your intentions.

The best way to get through these tests (and also to infuse flirting into the conversation) is to agree and exaggerate.

This is far better than what most guys do, which is to try and prove themselves. That's because it shows you have a sense of humor and don't take yourself too seriously.

Here are some examples of what it looks like to agree and exaggerate:

Her: "I'm sure you say that to every girl..."

You: "Damn it, you're right. Usually they don't catch on though. I must be off my game today."

-

Her: "You know I'm not sleeping with you tonight, right?"
You: "Obviously. Sex is always better on the second date anyway."

-

Her: "I'm too old for you..."
You: "Oh, I know. I'm just a boy trying to find his place in this big world. I'm no match for a sexy, mature girl like yourself."

Positioning Yourself as the Prize

Remember the "She's into me," mindset from the first section of this book?

Well, this is basically the verbalization of that mindset.

Here, you occasionally insinuate that she's hitting on you or trying to seduce you. You do this by twisting her words and making it seem like she's trying to turn you on.

In this way, you position yourself as the prize and position her as the pursuer.

Here are a few examples:

Her: "I love bikinis!"

You: "Don't try to make me think of you in a bikini."

-

Her: [Accidently grazes your elbow]

You: "Are you trying to seduce me?"

-

You: "I live around the corner. We can go to my place for a drink, but only if you promise not to try anything."

Keep in mind: when flirting, it's important to maintain at least a slight smile and good eye contact. This keeps the vibe fun, and let's her know that you're being playful.

Action Tip: Use one of these flirting techniques in your next conversation with a girl.

How to Tease Her the Right Way

Teasing is another conversational key to successful flirting.

If you aren't teasing girls the right way, you're probably missing out on A LOT of opportunities.

What's worse, when you tease her the wrong way, you risk:

- Offending her

- Making her feel insecure

- Hurting her

- And overall causing her to dislike you

These are all things women don't soon forget…

(She still may laugh at these teases, but it'll sting, and she'll probably close up.)

The problem is, guys have misconceptions about what it means to tease women. Part of this stems from the thinking that "you need to be a jerk" to attract women, and part of it stems from general social inexperience.

But teasing is essential to a flirty, fun conversation that attracts her to you. It's also important for separating you from the pathetic "nice guys" who constantly try to kiss her ass and please her.

For me, teasing has always been a bit natural. That's because my dad is a comedian, and I was lucky enough to attend many of his shows. He works the crowd like Don Rickles, and teases everybody.

I began to internalize his style and slowly refine it. His delivery of teases is powerful and always draws laughs. You can see a quick clip of his comedy here: https://www.youtube.com/watch?v=vHlT13QP5U8

With this in mind, let's break down teasing into two steps: 1) what to avoid and 2) how to tease her the right way.

The Wrong Teasing: What to Avoid

Sensitive Topics Don't tease girls about sensitive topics that may offend them. You should inherently know what most of these topics are. Topics like:
- Physical features

- Fashion/style

- Social skills
- Intelligence
- Family

She's likely to take these types of teases as insults. S

o you'd want to avoid making jokes like, "I can't believe you thought that was true. What's going on in that head up there?" (insinuating she's dumb).

And you definitely, DEFINITELY, want to avoid making any sort of jokes about her weight. There's no quicker way to get yourself in the doghouse with a woman.

Critiquing Her

Don't tease her about things you don't like about her. That's an easy way to come off as passive-aggressive. For example, let's say you don't like the fact that she doesn't eat healthy....

It'd be kind of a mean thing to say, "You look pretty good for someone addicted to sugary foods..."

Nobody likes hearing that they suck. What's worse, she'll feel like you're judging her. And if you're judging her about one thing, what's to say you're not going to judge her for something like sleeping with you quickly? In short, this is a good way to ruin your chances make her feel bad.

Putting Her Down

You also don't want to make her feel bad for what she likes and dislikes. This puts her in an awkward position because she feels bad for being who she is. And if she can't feel like she can be herself around you, you're as good as done.

For example:

"What's your favorite TV show? And please don't say The Bachelor."

Teasing the Whole Time/Being a Clown

You should weave teasing into the conversation – but the conversation shouldn't be one long tease. Women will start to question why you're never serious. They'll feel like you're trying to hide something behind your mask of constant humor. Instead, try to strike a balance between teasing and having meaningful conversation.

Making Fun of Yourself

Self-deprecating humor can be funny around your boys, and it might draw a laugh from her – but it usually won't help you get a date. Things like making fun of your weight, your difficulties with women, etc. A lot of comics do this all the time.

But when it comes to flirting and teasing women, self-deprecation usually isn't worth the laugh.

How to Tease Her the Right Way

Now you know what to avoid. But you still need to know what to do right. You can use these techniques to tease women better than the majority of men (and she'll love you for it).

Absurdify

Absurdifying is the art of taking a normal topic and making it a little ridiculous. This is a fun and playful way to tease her, and one of my personal go-to's. It also makes the conversation more intriguing because it's less predictable.

For example:

Her: "I'm from Pennsylvania."

You: "Nice, I love Pennsylvania. Are you a city girl or did you come straight out of Amish country?"

She has to qualify herself as to why she's not from Amish country, which is bound to be a ridiculous and fun conversation.

Bring Yourself Into It

When you include yourself, it creates a fun, "we're in this together" type of vibe, which is important for building a connection.

My dad does a great job of this in his comedy routine (in the video at the beginning of this chapter). Give it another watch and see how he includes himself in all the teases, so both the crowd and the people he's teasing can feel good and get a laugh.

And here's a conversational example: "Oh, so you're a psych major? You're probably reading my mind right now, aren't you? I'm on to you."

Stereotype Her in a Fun Way

Here, you basically play off the stereotypes of something she tells you. For example: "Oh, you're a country girl? So what do you do when you're not square dancing or listening to "Chicken Fried"?

"A Boston girl, huh? So you're not familiar with the letter "r"?"

Challenge Her

You can challenge her with something like a "thumb wrestle". If you're on the dance floor, you can give her a playful "hip bump," then step back and jokingly challenge her to a dance off (this is a great way to attract women at the nightclub).

Mock Her

This is especially great if she has an accent and/or says a word particularly weird. You can exaggerate her accent or mimic the particular word.

For example, a lot of Spanish speaking girls have trouble saying the "i" in words like "pill", "give", and "pick". They pronounce it like an "e" (i.e. pill = peel). So I always have a good time mocking their pronunciations of these words.

Playfully Disagree With Her

Playfully disagree with her about something and turn your back.

For example:

"I can't believe you don't watch Game of Thrones. We can't be friends anymore," and then turn your back and pretend to walk away for a few steps.

Accuse Her of Hitting on You

This is funny, but also reverses the roles. She's used to being the prize, but when you accuse her of hitting on you, you flip the script. Now she's the one trying to seduce you.

For example:

"Are you hitting on me right now?

"I see what you're trying to do. But I'm not that easy!"

"I saw you checking me out over there. I'm not a piece of meat you know."

"Okay, we can go back to my place. But only if you promise not to try anything."

Teasing is all about being self-amused and lighthearted. You should be enjoying yourself, and not aiming to impress her with the quality of your jokes. Teasing should help you connect with her and also express your personality.
One more note – don't be afraid to straddle the line with the occasional crude joke or sexual innuendo. It's okay to take risks, and fortune favors the bold.

Action Tip: Choose at least one of these teasing techniques and use it in your next conversation with a girl. It's okay if you mess it up the first few times – it takes a little practice!

Flirting Without Your Words

You've learned how to flirt with your words. But that's not all that goes on in a conversation. There's always a non-verbal level. And if you don't know how to communicate on that level, your flirting will fall flat.

So, what goes on in that non-verbal level? How do you master it?

That's what this chapter is all about.

We'll go through each level of non-verbal flirting so you can make your flirting sexy.

Let's get started.

Sexy Eye Contact

We've covered eye contact a bit already in this book. But here are a few ways you can use it in for sexy flirting:

The "triangle gazing routine" – You look at her eyes, then down to her mouth, then back up to her eyes – in a triangle formation. This is a great way to show interest in her.

Bedroom eyes – Lower your eyelids and have a sort of dreamy expression. This is easiest when you focus on what you like about her. When you're basking in her feminine energy and beauty, it's easy to have this sort of dreamy, satisfied look.

Move your eyes slowly – Avoid darting your eyes back and forth. When you move your eyes, move them slowly. This conveys more confidence and control.

Match her gaze – When she's speaking, you should be looking into her eyes about 90-95% of the time. Only look away when she's looking away. Sometimes, girls will make less eye contact because they're nervous or simply uncomfortable with eye contact. In this case, you should look away about 25% of the time that she looks away.

The more you interact with women and practice these eye contact techniques, the more comfortable (and better) you'll be with sexy eye contact. So, give these a try.

Close Proximity

How close are you when you flirt with women?

As a general rule, the closer, the better.

You see, as you decrease the distance between you, the level of intention and intimacy increases. So, how do you close the proximity? There are a few easy ways to do this... *Always sit next to her on a date* – When you're having drinks with her for a date, always aim to sit at the bar with her. This way, you can sit next to her rather than across from her.

Talk in her ear, and bounce out – This is key, especially in loud venues. Lean in and speak into her ear while lightly touching her elbow. Then, when you're done talking, bounce out to hear her response. In doing so, you close the proximity, but also give her room to breathe. Then, the next time you lean in and talk in her ear, it's even more powerful.

Face her head-on instead of at an angle – When you face her head on, it's more intimate and flirtatious.

Physical Touch

Physical touch is crucial to making a connection, and it's also crucial to sexy flirting.

You should be touching her early and often.

The quicker you touch her, the quicker you assert yourself as both a dominant and sexual man who goes for what he wants.

But you need to use physical touch the right way.

Here's how:

Touch her in the right places – The best places to touch her are her elbow, upper arm, and the small of her back. You can touch her elbow and upper arm when you're joking with her in conversation or leaning in to speak into her ear. And you can touch the small of her back when you're showing her something with your hand, or leading her (i.e. walking with her to the bar).

Touch her early in the conversation – The easiest way to do this is with a handshake (or a hug) and an introduction. By touching her immediately, you set a flirtatious tone for the conversation. You've broken the "physical barrier".

Touch her at the right moments – For example, touch her when the two of you are laughing or when she's agreeing with you. That way, she'll associate positive feelings with your touch.

Don't draw attention to the touch – I once coached a guy who would look at his hand every time he touched a girl, or even so much as went in for a handshake. It freaked women out, because it seemed so unnatural. Whatever you do, make sure you DON'T look at your hand when you touch her.

Make sure you're close to her – There are few things more awkward than reaching out a few feet to touch a girl. The closer you are, the better.
Hold her hand when walking through a crowd – For example, lets say you're at the bar with her, and want to go for a drink. You can say, "Let's go

for a drink at the bar," then take her hand and lead her through the crowd.

Ask about her jewelry – Notice that she has some cool jewelry on her wrist? Lightly take her hand, and ask her the meaning of the jewelry.

***

Alright, so to recap, here are the 3 keys to sexy nonverbal flirting:

1. Sexy eye contact

2. Close proximity

3. Physical touch

When you combine these non-verbal techniques with the verbal techniques, you'll be flirting like a Casanova.

Action Tip: Use at least one of these non-verbal flirting techniques in your next conversation with a woman.

Part IV: Connect

Get Her Talking

You now have a basic framework for:

- Getting through your fear of approaching new women

- Starting a conversation

- Making a great first impression

- Flirting

- Continuing the conversation and getting her number

These elements are great, especially for shorter conversations. But what about when you're on a date, at the bar, or even in a relationship? You need to know how to have longer conversations and connect with women on a deeper level.

And to do that, you need to get her talking. You see, the more she talks about herself, the more she'll feel connected to you.

In this section, you'll learn how to do exactly that: get past small talk and get her talking about herself. Let's get started...

How to Get Past Small Talk and Connect With Her

Small talk.

It's the baron wasteland of conversation that seems so hard to get past. When you're in small talk, you're basically treading water. You're staying afloat, but you're not getting anywhere.

Even if you start the conversation well, you still need to get to know the other person. You still need to get beyond the basic "stuff" like where they're from and what they think of the weather.

You need to stir up some emotions.

But this can seem like a daunting task. And that task can seem even more daunting when your conversational counterpart is a beautiful woman. Your mind either draws a blank, or starts running a million miles per minute.

"What do I say? What if she thinks I'm stupid? What if she gets bored?"

That's when you fall into "interview mode" where you're asking basic questions that require a one or two word answer. The result? The conversation stalls out. And then you beat yourself up over it.

Here's what happens when you constantly engage in small talk:

- Women will flake on you A LOT

- Women won't remember you

- Women won't feel like they know you

- And worse, they won't feel like you understand them

If this sounds familiar to you – don't sweat it. It happens to every guy at one point or another. But there's an easier way to make the conversation flow…and it doesn't require you to employ a bunch of intricate conversation tricks. Hell, you don't even have to talk that much.

In fact, if you're doing it right, the girl will be talking more than you.

So, how can you beat small talk, make the conversation flow, and build a connection?

It's a combination of the following:

- Asking the right questions

- Listening and relating

- Avoiding common conversation mistakes

We'll cover each one in this chapter.

Asking the Right Questions

A few simple, pointed questions can draw her interest, open the conversation, and help you plow past small talk.

Think about it – when you're in "interview mode", she doesn't even have to think. She can basically respond on autopilot because she's had that same type of conversation hundreds of times.

But when you ask the right questions, you cause a pattern-interrupt. All of the sudden, she has to think. She has to ponder her motivations and actually feel things. Beyond that, you also allow her to talk about herself, her passions, and her motivations. This instantly breaks you out of small talk.

I will give you some powerful (and simple) questions to point you in the right direction, but more importantly, you'll learn how to structure your questions, so that you can further the conversation instead of lead it to a dead-end of awkward silence.

If you do this right, you'll be able to transform women from being cold and closed off, to warm and open.

Sidenote: These questions, along with the question structure, are relevant to any conversation, whether you're chatting with the hottie at the bar, a networking event, or any random situations you find yourself in.

Why Questions Are Important

This is counterintuitive, but when you prompt people to tell you about themselves, they actually perceive you as more interesting...even if they barely know anything about you.

Scientists have found that talking about ourselves activates the same pleasure centers of the brain that are associated with food and money. [1]

And the best way to prompt people to do so is to ask the right questions...

...Questions that allow the other person to open up to you and talk about the stuff they really care about.

By asking the right questions and taking the time to listen to their responses, you'll get paid back tenfold. They undoubtedly will reciprocate and show a lot of interest in your life.

How to Structure Your Questions

There are two main types of questions we'll deal with here: Short-answer questions, and open-ended questions.

Short-Answer Questions: Ask too many of these types of questions in a row, and you'll find yourself deep in "interview mode" on a conversational path that leads to nowhere. These are the questions that only require a one-word response, like:

- "Where did you go to school?"
- "What do you do?"
- "Where are you from?"

Now, it's okay to ask these types of questions, especially at the beginning of the conversation. In fact, it's almost necessary. But, unless you follow up with open-ended questions, the conversation will fall flat.

Open-Ended Questions: These questions require a deeper and more extended response. More than yes/no, or one word. These are your money questions. If you can master these, you'll be able to open up almost any conversation. Here's how you can mix these in with short-answer questions:

You: "What do you do?" (short-answer question)

Her: "I'm a lawyer."

You: "Cool cool. How did you get into that?" (open-ended question)
Her: "Well, my dad was a lawyer and ever since I was a kid, I...[blah blah blah]"

You: "Oh wow, that's awesome. What do you like about it?" (open-ended question)

Her: "Well, I really like helping people and..."

The key with open-ended questions is that you need to dig a little deeper. For example, instead of asking "Did you like it?", ask "What did you like about it?"

And remember: You need to balance short-answer questions with open-ended questions.
Here are some powerful open-ended questions to ask:

- What do you like about your job?

- What was it like growing up there (where they grew up)?

- If you could wake up anywhere in the world tomorrow, where would it be?

- What's your dream job?

- Why are you doing X instead of doing Y?

Listening and Relating

Questions are important – but you shouldn't just rattle question after question at her – even if they're good, open-ended questions.

This is a big mistake guys make. Instead of actively listening to a woman, they nod along with a blank stare, or wait for her to shut up so they can say what they want.

When you don't actively listen, it makes the girl feel like you don't understand her. In fact, she feels like you don't even really care.

So, what should you do instead?

When she's telling you about herself, actively listen to her, and relate back to her responses. Provide some sort of feedback, even if it's as simple as repeating back what she said.

For example, let's say that she tells you about how she loved studying abroad in Spain.

You could respond with something like: "That's awesome that you lived in Spain! I've been learning Spanish – Spain is on my list of places to go!"

She might say, "That's great! I definitely recommend it."

To which you could say, "Great…so, what made you want to live in Spain?"

This shows that you listen and you "get it," and also allows her to reveal her motivations to you (a strong emotional topic).

Plus, it shows that you're interested in her as well. This eases the social pressure and makes her feel like you're on her side.

Here's another example…

You: "What do you do?"

Her: "I'm an architect"

You: "Ah that's awesome. One of my favorite parts of walking through NYC is looking at all the beautiful architecture. It's crazy how the city is filled with so many beautiful buildings. You must get some inspiration from them, right?"

Her: "Yeah! The buildings here are awesome."

You: "For sure… So tell me, what made you want to get into architecture?"

Her: "Well, I've always loved creating things. Ever since I was a kid, I dreamed of designing a building that would be part of the NYC skyline."

You: "Oh yeah? It sounds like you're doing something you're really passionate about! So what kind of building would it be?"

Avoiding Common Conversation Mistakes

The more you get past small talk, the more risks you will take in conversations, and the more potential mistakes you will be exposed to.

That's why I'm going to highlight a few "mistakes" for you to be aware of. These mistakes will make you come across as an asshole and/or make the girl feel like you don't "get" her.

And so, I'd like to help you avoid them.

These mistakes are all based on a psychological concept known as "the other."

What is "the other?" Well, do you ever feel like there are people who "get you", and then, there's everybody else? You know, people who just understand you and your lifestyle…and then the people who can't begin to relate to you?

That's what I mean by "the other."

You see, we have a tendency to view everything in the world (including other human beings) as being either the "same" as ourselves, or "other" (i.e. "with us" or "against us").

And rightfully so. This "same vs. other" concept protects us from potential threats and helps us stick with the people who understand us best and are most likely to support us.

But when it comes to seducing and connecting with women, it's where many guys destroy their chances. That's because many guys are great at positioning themselves as "the other", and not very good at showing how they are "the same". But in order to emotionally connect with women, you need to help women see you as the "same" as them.
So the goal of highlighting these mistakes is to help you stop doing things that make women view you as "the other" so you can make connections with them.

Mistake #1: Stating Contentious Opinions

Let's say you love to meditate.

You're on a date with a girl, and she says, "You know what I can't stand? People who meditate. They just sit there doing nothing and claim that it clears their mind. What a waste of time."

How would you feel? Probably much less connected to her, right? T

his is exactly what you want to avoid doing to her. There's really no reason for stating contentious opinions and it only puts you at risk of ruining the connection.

Solution #1: Be Non-Judgmental and Focus on Commonalities

When you're trying to connect with a girl, it's best to avoid arguments and contention. These will put you in the "other" category faster than anything else.

If you hate 9-5 jobs and cubicles, but she works a desk job that she enjoys, it's probably not a great idea to go on about how much you despise conventional jobs (I've made this mistake many times).

Instead, focus on things you can easily relate to each other on, like interests and hobbies. For example, maybe you both like to travel, read, or have a favorite Netflix show in common.

(Note: It is okay to disagree with girls without being contentious. Just avoid making it a big deal and a major part of the conversation.)

Mistake #2: Getting Married to a Conversation Topic

You know that feeling when you're done talking about something, but your conversation counterpart keeps bringing it back up? It's like, "Bro, I know you like working out, but I don't want to talk about the nuances of deadlifts for 3 hours."

Every conversation topic has a lifespan, and if you try to milk the topic past its lifespan, you'll annoy people (and turn women off).

You may be tempted to do this because you'll naturally be more comfortable with certain conversation topics. For example, if you enjoy working out, you'll be comfortable talking about lifting weights. But you can't allow yourself to keep falling back to this topic – you must keep the conversation flowing...

Solution #2: Weave in Multiple Topics

A rich conversation weaves through multiple topics.

It's okay to change the subject, even if you haven't said everything you feel like you need to say about a topic. But when you keep reverting back to a conversation topic, it signals to women that you have low social intelligence and also that you're not a very well rounded man.

If you feel like you want to keep coming back to a "dead" topic, stop yourself, and ask a good question to push the conversation forward (like, "What are you passionate about?").

It's also important to keep the conversation focused on more emotional topics.

Here are some emotional topics for you to dive into:

- Her dreams
- Her experiences
- What she loves to do
- What she is passionate about
- What her motivations are

(We'll talk more about these emotional conversation topics in the next chapter.)

Mistake #3: Talking Too Much About Yourself

A friend told me she went on a Tinder date the other day with a doctor. He was handsome, successful, and rich. Everything a woman wants, right?

But within an hour, she had her friend call her and give the "sick grandma excuse" so she could escape this terrible date.

(The "sick grandma excuse" is when a girl has her friend call her 30 minutes to an hour into a date. If she's having fun, she'll hang up and stay on the date. If she's not, she'll say, "My mom just called. My grandma is sick and I have to go see her.")

So, what happened?

The guy ranted and raved about himself, his success, and his importance. She felt like she couldn't be herself around him, like he was constantly judging her.
He positioned himself as "the other" right from the beginning and it killed any attraction and hope for a connection.

Solution #3: Focus the Conversation on the Girl

You don't have to say that much about yourself, especially in your first conversation. In fact, you can tell her very little while having her open up and tell her almost everything about herself.

Remember: Talking about ourselves activates the same pleasure centers of the brain that are associated with food and money. The more she talks about herself, the more connected she'll feel to you.

Action Tip #1: Write down 5 open-ended questions. Focus them around emotional topics like we talked about here. For example, "What are you most passionate about?"

Action tip #2: Write down the conversation mistake (from the list above) that you feel like you're most guilty of. This will help you be more aware of it and avoid it in the future.

Reference:

1. Tamir, Diana I., and Jason P. Mitchell. "Disclosing information about the self is intrinsically rewarding." *Proceedings of the National Academy of Sciences* 109.21 (2012): 8038-8043.

5 Go-To Conversation Topics for Connecting

Remember: The more she talks about herself, the more connected she'll feel to you.

And in order to truly get her to talk about herself, you need to infuse emotional topics into the conversation.

Sure, it's nice to talk about the new club downtown, or how it sucks when it's raining outside, but those are conversations she can have with anyone. You want to move to topics that aren't universally relatable for everyone. That's how real connections are formed, and that's what this chapter is all about…

(Note: It's best to weave these topics into conversation. Don't formulaically cycle through them like a robot. Allow the conversation to flow and evolve. Also, try to relate back to her responses with something relevant from your own life. This shows her that you "get her" and that you're actually interested and paying attention.)

With this in mind, here are 5 go-to conversation topics that make it easy to talk and connect with women…

1. Her Experiences

Perhaps you've both gone scuba diving, or traveled to Vietnam. Or perhaps she quit her job and moved to a beach town to become a whale shark tour guide.

We've all had memorable experiences – good and bad, uplifting and scary. Experiences are tied to emotions – we're always feeling "stuff" when we go through them. That's why they're such a great topic. They can lead to amazing stories and tons of emotions, as well as unique ways to relate to each other.

Here are some questions that can get you to this topic:

- "What made you want to come to this city?"

- "What was your last big adventure?"

- "Where is your favorite place you've traveled?"

Once you get her talking about this, you can dive deeper and ask questions like:

- "How did it feel when you did X?"

- "What was it like to do X?"

When you ask these types of questions, you'll tap into the emotions she felt when she had those experiences.

2. Her Dreams

What does she really want to do with her life? What are her biggest aspirations?

Everybody thinks about their dreams – but not everybody gets to talk about those dreams. That's because most people never think to ask them.

But given the opportunity, most people would love to talk about their dreams and aspirations. That's why it brings up all sorts of good and hopeful emotions.

Here are some questions that can get you to this topic:

- "What's something you've always wanted to do?"

- "What's something you want to achieve this year?"

Once you get her talking about this, you can dive deeper and ask questions like:

- "How would it feel to do that?"

- "How would your life change if you accomplish that?"

3. What She Loves to Do

What do you love to do? Think about it for a minute...

No, really. Do it right now.

Did you think about it? Okay, good...

How did it feel? You probably pictured yourself doing those things, and you probably felt similar emotions as when you did them, right?

For me, I love performing on stage. Every time I think about it, I picture my past performances when there were huge crowds cheering for me, and I was killing it. It brings up a feeling of excitement.

When women talk about the things they love to do, the same thing happens. They feel those good emotions, and they associate those good emotions to being around you.

Here are some questions that can get you to this topic:
Here are sine questions that can get you to this topic:

- "What do you absolutely love to do?"

- "What kind of activities set you on fire and get you excited?"

- "What kinds of things make you laugh the hardest?"

Once you get her talking about this, you can dive deeper and ask questions like:

- "What do you love about X?"

- "How do you feel when you do X?"

4. Her Passions

What passions drive her?

Maybe she loves traveling, or perhaps she's extremely passionate about volunteering.

Her passions are another highly emotional topic. People love talking about them. What's more, a woman's passions can tell you a lot about her – as well as give you a glimpse into whether you are a good fit for each other.

You may find that you have similar passions, which makes it very easy to relate and connect with her.

Here is a question that can get you to this topic: "What are you most passionate about?"

Once you get her talking about this, you can dive deeper and ask questions like:

- "What makes you passionate about X?"

- "How do you feel when you're following that passion?"

5. Her Motivations

Why does she want the things she wants? What are her true motivations? Most men never dig this deep...

They ask questions like, "What do you do?" She responds with something like, "Oh I'm a lawyer." He follows up with, "Cool! Do you like it?" to which she responds, "It's okay, and what about you?"

That's the foundation of a boring, polite, platonic conversation. And that's exactly what you DON'T want...

Instead, try to figure out exactly why she wants the things she wants. When you do this from a place of curiosity, it shows that you're interested and not afraid to dive a little deeper. It's quite the pattern interrupt but that's a good thing.

Here are some questions that can get you to this topic:

- "What made you want to get into that?" (If she's discussing her career or college major)

- "What made you do that?" (If she's discussing a story or a choice she's made)

Once you get her talking about this, you can dive deeper and ask questions like:

- "Now that you're doing X, how do you feel about it?"

- "Why did you want to accomplish X?"

***

The more you dive into these kinds of emotional topics, the easier you'll connect with women. You'll stop having polite, "just friends" conversations. What's more, you'll start sparking attraction with your words, and find that A LOT more women are "into you."

So, use these with caution, and break them out when you genuinely want to connect with women.

Action Tip: Choose at least one of these conversation topics and use them in your next conversation with a woman.

Part V: Captivate

How to Talk About Yourself in an Attractive Way

"So you know all this about me... I want to know more about you!" she tells you...

"Well, what do you want to know," you say with sly smile.

"I don't know. What do you do? What's your story?" she responds...

"Well..."

What are you going to say? How are you going to talk about yourself?

While it's best to get her talking about herself, as well as create a fun, flirty conversation, at some point she'll want to know about you.

Whether she asks you for your story or you relate things about your life throughout the conversation – you need to know how to talk about yourself in an attractive way.

But most men do this all wrong. How? In a few ways...

First, they focus on facts and stats over emotions.

They say things like, "Well, I've been to 5 countries, I have THIS car, I run a successful business, I'm a doctor, etc."

All of these things sound nice. Impressive, even. But there's one big problem... Women don't connect with facts and stats. They connect with emotions.

And the way to communicate emotionally is to tell better stories and communicate good qualities. But...

Most men also tell terrible stories...

They infuse their stories with "humble brags" and don't talk about the emotions involved. Instead, they just convey the facts and talk about what happened. What's worse, they don't involve the other person in the story at all. They talk AT the woman the whole time, instead of WITH her.

But even when men do tell good stories, they struggle to...

Convey the right qualities about themselves...

You see, one of the keys to talking about yourself is to convey attractive qualities. If you don't know the right qualities to convey and how to convey them, you risk killing the connection and making dumb mistakes.

Speaking of mistakes, the other big one men make when talking about themselves is that **they give away too much too quickly.**

You don't need to be a completely open book, especially when you just meet somebody.

We've all met that person who seems to give it all up right away. They go into their life story without even being prompted. It's annoying, right?

It's better to hold a little back and be intriguing.

Okay okay, how's all this sound? At this point, you may be a little overwhelmed. "I'm making a lot of these mistakes right now!" you may be thinking…

That's okay though. That's why you have this book – to learn how to avoid the common mistakes and communicate more effectively (and attractively). And that's what you're going to learn throughout this chapter and this section.

When you talk about yourself in an attractive way, you can literally "flip" the attraction switch in a woman's mind. If she wasn't into you before, you can open her up to the idea of being with you. And if she was already interested in you, you can keep building that interest to the point where she's open to taking the next step with you (perhaps leaving the bar and going home with you).

So, how do you talk about yourself in an attractive way?

There are a few elements to this:

1) Understand the purpose of talking about yourself

2) Highlight sexy qualities about yourself

3) Bait her

4) Follow the proper etiquette

We'll go into each of these 4 elements so you can start talking about yourself in an attractive way.

Step #1: Understand the Purpose of Talking About Yourself

The purpose is actually quite simple: To quickly excite and intrigue her and then turn the conversation back over to her.
You're not trying to tell her your life story or convince her why you're the perfect man for her. You're not trying to list out all of your impressive accolades.

Just excite her, intrigue her, and get her talking about herself again.

Step #2: Highlight Sexy Qualities About Yourself

How do you excite and intrigue her? It starts by highlighting the right qualities about yourself.

Most men THINK that women are attracted to:

- A good job

- Lots of money

- Good looks

While these things are good to have, they aren't at the root of attraction. In other words, they aren't enough.

(Just ask the guy who worked his whole life to make a lot of money, assuming that women would love him for it. Only to realize later that having a lot of money doesn't do the trick...)

So when you try to convey these qualities in conversation, you just seem like you're trying to impress the girl.

But what qualities are women actually attracted to?

There are 3 main qualities you should keep in mind:

1) Dominance

2) Sociability

3) Altruism

So, why these qualities? Let's start with dominance…

Think about how a stereotypical "nice guy" interacts with women. He plays it safe, waits for overwhelming signs of attraction before making a move, and doesn't get laid all that much (if at all). For women, being with this kind of man is a chore.

Now, think of how a dominant man acts. Women are an abundant resource for him, so he doesn't put them on a pedestal. He knows what he wants in life, and goes for it unapologetically. What's more, women don't have to worry about much when they're with a dominant man – they can relax, knowing that he'll do the leading and make her feel good emotions.

Dominance, then, is an indicator that a guy is successful with women and has control of his life. And so, it is very attractive to women.

So, how can you convey dominance in conversation? Here are some examples you could talk about:

- A time where you achieved something you once thought was impossible

- How you took charge of a situation even though you were unsure of the outcome

- A time where you successfully led a group of people

Here's a quick example:

"I love creating art, but everybody told me, 'You can never succeed in that profession. It's a poor man's game.' This only motivated me more – I wanted to prove everybody wrong and make it happen. So, I buckled down and kept improving my painting skills, and I read a few books about marketing. Within 2 months, I had sold my first painting for a nice sum. And all those haters had nothing to say!"

Now, let's go over sociability.

A woman wants to feel like she can bring you around her friends without having to worry that you could potentially creep them out or do something weird.

What's more, sociability signals that you're a cool, confident guy who can talk to anybody.

The sociable guy communicates with people with ease, has a big social circle, and is well connected. This signals that he's successful with women, and has abundance in his life (with women, friends, and money).

So, how can you convey sociability in conversation? Here are some examples you could talk about:

- A time where you hung out with a group of friends and had fun
- A time where you connected with someone you looked up to
- A time where you introduced two groups of friends to each other

And finally, let's talk about altruism.

A study by Evolutionary Psychology found that, at least for serious relationships, women value altruism over good looks. In other words, they're more likely to choose an average-looking altruistic man than an attractive but non-altruistic one. [1] Altruistic behaviors are those intended to help other people. When you're altruistic, you're concerned about the rights, feelings, and welfare of other people.

Some behaviors you'd associate with altruism are feeling empathy, as well as acting in ways that benefit other people.

Again, let's look at this through a nice guy lens. The typical "nice guy" is a little bitter towards women. Most of his actions are meant to get something from other people (especially women) without much of a care for how those other people feel. And so, he's not very altruistic.

Now, let's look at the altruistic man. This guy doesn't do everything with an ulterior motive. He does altruistic and selfless things as an end in themselves.

And so, altruism indicates that a man is genuine, caring, and not looking to "get" something from everybody he interacts with.

So, how can you convey altruism in conversation? Here are some examples you could talk about:

- A time where you helped somebody less fortunate

- A time where you did some volunteer work

- A time where you helped a friend accomplish something

Here's a quick example of altruism:

"Living in Medellin, Colombia was a ton of fun. We had some awesome parties and met tons of cool people. But one of the most memorable parts was taking a trip up to poorest section of the city and handing out shoes to the little kids. Have you ever done volunteer work by the way? This was my first time. Anyway, these kids either had no shoes, or extremely beaten-up shoes. So, seeing the looks on their faces when we handed them some brand new shoes was amazing. The whole experience really put everything into perspective."

So, dominance, sociability, and altruism. If you can convey these qualities, you can come off very attractive to women.

Aside from these three main qualities, there are some secondary qualities you should highlight as well.

-Adventurousness. Women love spontaneous men. They want the kind of guy who's going to make them feel alive, challenge them, and excite them. Not the kind of guy they can easily predict.

-Appreciation of Beauty. Men who appreciate beauty usually genuinely love women. What's more, they also tend to enjoy good intimacy.

-Sense of humor. Women like a man who can make her laugh and make light of situations, versus those men who take themselves too seriously.

Step #3: Bait Her

When it comes to talking about yourself, it's always more powerful when she asks you about something than when you straight up tell her. We all know those people who drone on about themselves without prompting. You don't want to be that guy.

It's far better if she has to dig a little bit to discover more about you.

That's where baiting comes into play.

Baiting causes women to put effort into finding out who you are. It makes you seem A LOT more interesting, and even adds a bit of mystery.

We're going to discuss 3 specifics forms of baiting – you'll want to infuse all of these into your conversations.

Baiting technique 1: Make an intriguing statement.

Let's say a girl asks what you do…

You could say, "I'm a stockbroker…I also enjoy dancing."

Okay, that's fine – but it doesn't give her much to work with. Plus, it paints you as a bit of a boring, typical guy. Now, let's look at how you can answer this in a more intriguing way…

When she asks what you do, you can say, "I love to lay down the moves on the salsa dance floor, but I also analyze businesses."

This is short on details, and it gives her a lot to work with. She'll be curious about how you learned to dance salsa, as well as what you mean by "analyze businesses." This will instantly make you appear more intriguing.

Here's another example…

Let's say she asks you what you like to do…

You could say, "I like reading books and learning in general."

Again, a bit of a boring statement. Now, let's add some baiting into it…

"I love learning and improving. I feel like if you're not stretching your comfort zone and feeling a little stupid some of the time, you're not really living."

Now she's thinking, "What does he mean by 'learning?' And how has he stretched his comfort zone?"

She'll want to dig deeper and learn more about you.

Baiting technique 2: Reciprocity

In his groundbreaking book *Influence*, author Robert Cialdini discusses the 6 key influence tactics of psychology and persuasion. One of the most powerful of those tactics is reciprocity.

What is reciprocity? Well, as humans, we generally aim to return favors and pay people back when they've given us something. We have the strong urge to reciprocate. For example, have you ever asked to sample more than a couple of flavors at an ice cream shop? After you've sampled a few, do you feel compelled to buy something, even if you don't really have the strong urge to eat anymore ice cream?

That's reciprocity in action. You can use this reciprocity tactic to bait her in conversations. How?

When you dive deep on a particular topic about her life, she'll feel compelled to ask you about that same topic.

For example, let's say you've used the question structure from part 3, and she's told you about her career, what made her get into it, what she likes about it, etc. Maybe the two of you have spent 3-5 minutes or more discussing it.

She's going to feel a lot of social pressure to reciprocate and ask what you do. At that point, you can use the first baiting technique to keep her intrigued and interested.

Baiting technique 3: The open loop

Have you ever watched the hit series *Game of Thrones*? They end every episode with a huge open loop that gets you excited and interested in the next episode or the next season. That open loop stays on the back of your mind all week until the next episode airs. It's powerful stuff.

You can also use these open loops in conversation.

For example, let's say she's talking about travel...

Her: "I traveled abroad in Spain when I was in college. It was a great experience."

You: "Spain is one of my favorite countries! What did you think about the culture?"

Her: "It was amazing! So much different than here. The tapas were incredible and the people were so stylish. What'd you think of Spain? And what other countries have you been to?"

Can you spot the open loop in this example? If you missed it, here it is:

"Spain is **one of my favorite countries**! What did you think about the culture?

By telling her Spain is one of your favorite countries, you indirectly signal that you've been to other countries (and you have the quality of adventurousness). But then, you continue on with an open-ended question.

You've created an open loop in her mind, because she'll be curious about what other countries you've been to. And by following it up with an open-ended question about her, you do it in a socially savvy way. I

f you just said, "Spain is one of my favorite countries!" you'd signal, "Yeah, look at how cool I am, I travel so much." But instead, you put the open loop in as kind of a throwaway detail on your way to discovering more about her. You don't focus on it, and so it doesn't come across like you're trying to impress her.

And yet, it still plants the question in her mind, "What other countries has he been to?" and lays the groundwork for a deeper conversation.

Step #4: Follow the Proper Etiquette

It's not enough to know how to highlight the right qualities about yourself and bait women. You must also follow the proper etiquette for talking about yourself.

Otherwise you risk talking about yourself too much, coming across as unattainable, and damaging the connection.

In terms of "talk about yourself" etiquette, there are 3 rules you should follow...

Rule 1: Don't make the conversation all about you

Remember: The more she talks about herself, the more connected she'll feel to you.

So, she doesn't need to know that much about you to feel like she's connected to you.

With this in mind, you shouldn't be talking about yourself for the majority of the conversation. In fact, you should keep it to a minimum.

That way, she's the one talking about herself, qualifying herself to you, and really putting most of the effort in. All while you sit back, make some intriguing statements, tell a few pointed stories, and let the conversation flow.

How can you do this? After talking about yourself briefly, turn the conversation back over to her. You can do this by:

Asking her the same question she asked you. If you've just told her what you do, you can ask her what she does.

Include her in the conversation by infusing questions about your topic. If you're telling her a story about snorkeling, you could say something like, "I LOVE snorkeling – have you ever tried it?" to which she may launch into a tale about how she loves snorkeling too.

Ask her a random question. You can use this as your backup plan if you feel like the conversation topic has dried up. You simply ask her a random question like, "Where have you traveled to?"

Here's an example of turning the conversation back to her smoothly...

Her: "How'd you end up starting your own fitness blog?"

You: "Well, after I finished college I was pretty out of shape. One of the guys I worked with was passionate about fitness, and he got me into it. It completely enthralled me. I ended up quitting my office job to become a personal trainer, then I thought, "How can I help more people get in shape, rather than just a few clients a day?" That's why I started up my fitness blog a few years ago – to reach as many people as possible. It took a while to build traction, and a lot of people doubted me. At one point when my money was low, I even considered quitting and going back to a regular job. But I kept at it, and eventually I managed to get published on a few big sites. From there, it kept growing."

Her: "That's so interesting!"

You: "Yeah it's been quite the experience. It just seems like such a long journey when I reflect on it! What about you though – you said you wanted to get into photography when you were younger, but it never quite panned out. What stopped you from pursuing that?"

Here, you've built an interesting picture of yourself and made her curious. You haven't divulged all the details. Plus, you've given her a chance to talk even more about herself.

Rule 2: Know your "hero story"

Average is boring. Women like men who succeed in the face of adversity, overcome obstacles, and have purpose.
So, when you're talking about yourself, you want to convey these things.

That's where your "hero story" comes into play. As an example, you can look at the previous "hero story" about the fitness blog.

1) He started by talking about himself when he was younger and a goal that he had, but wasn't sure how to accomplish.

2) He mentioned a few obstacles along his way to success.

3) He talked about how he began to finally see some success.

4) He talked about his ultimate success (getting published on bigger sites and growing his blog)

This is the basic "hero story" format. We all have multiple hero stories. If you think a little bit, you can definitely come up with a few from your life.

Maybe it was the time you got the job (or promotion) you didn't think you could get, or the time you made the basketball team in high school against all odds. You can make any triumph into a hero story.

These "hero stories" show that you're not just any average schmuck. You're the type of guy who doesn't shrink in the face of a challenge – and women love that.

Rule 3: Make it playful

Don't paint yourself as "perfect". Instead, poke some fun at your mistakes, and show that you've struggled to get to your successes despite a few mishaps along the way. It wasn't all rainbows and unicorns.

You can also add in some light-hearted playfulness. For example, going back to the fitness blog guy, he could have joked, "Hell, back in college I barely even knew what a dumbbell was!"

Okay, so there you have it. You now know what to do to talk about yourself in an attractive way.

To recap:

Step #1: Understand the purpose of talking about yourself

Step #2: Highlight sexy qualities about yourself

Step #3: Bait her

Step #4: Follow the proper etiquette.

But how do you put all this together and infuse it into your conversations? One of the best ways to do it is through storytelling...

Luckily, you're about to learn how to tell a kick-ass story that hooks her in!

Reference:

1. Farrelly, Daniel, Paul Clemson and Melissa Guthrie. "Are Women's Mate Preferences for Altruism Also Influenced by Physical Attractiveness?" *Evolutionary Psychology* 14.1 (2016)

How to Tell a Kick-Ass Story That Hooks Her In

The music bumped and the ground shook below me. I looked around in awe.

I had just stepped into my first nightclub in Asia, after nearly 30 hours of travel. And I was scared.

I was with some of the guys from the entrepreneur group there. My friend had introduced me to them over some drinks and hookah earlier in the night. But that didn't do much to ease my comfort level.

Sure, I loved nightlife. But this was a whole different beast. I was sleep-deprived and surrounded by unfamiliar faces.

What's worse – I was thinking of the girl I had just left behind in Boston. Natalie. I'd never liked a girl as much as I liked her. We had an amazing two months together, but I had to leave her to embark on this journey, all the way across the globe to Vietnam.

Have you ever had to leave a girl prematurely like this? Maybe you know the feeling...

As I stood for a second, lost in thought, one of the guys from the entrepreneur group interrupted...

"Let's go approach some girls, bro!"

He was a hyper, 18-year-old dude who was already successful in business. I was not in the mood to approach girls, but he wouldn't take "no" for an answer.

After a few attempted conversations, I escaped to the bathroom. I walked back out to the dance floor, looked around one more time, and broke into a sweat.

The weird electronic music, the crazy environment, the foreign languages… It was all too much, too fast…

I couldn't take it…

***

We communicate best through stories. Stories are what hook us in and make us feel things.

And if you think about it, storytelling is key for most things involving people – whether it's teaching, writing, speaking, selling, leading, or attracting women…

A good story snaps people out of their boredom and captivates them. But good storytelling? That's hard to do – and very few people ever practice the skill. By the end of this chapter, though, you'll have all the tools you need to tell great stories.

So, what is good storytelling? Well, the "telling" part and the "story" part are two different beasts. You can have all the aspects that make a good story, but if you don't tell it well, it won't be a good story. You need both pieces.

And to top it off, you need to know how to tell it in a way that attracts women. We'll cover all the pieces in this chapter.

The first piece is the way you tell the story.

To tell a story well, you should have a handle on the most important aspect of good storytelling:

Tell the story as if you're living it.

You want to hold your listener's hand and walk her through every twist and turn, so that she's on the edge of her seat. How do you do that?

It's a combination of your tonality, facial expressions, and mood at each moment of your story. You want her to feel like you felt at the time – not like "it's already over and everything turned out okay."

Keep the sense of mystery alive. To see some examples of this in action, I recommend checking out comedians like John Mulaney, Bill Burr, and Eugene Mirman. These dudes know how to keep the mystery (and hilarity) going throughout their stories.

You can start with these clips by John Mulaney:

https://www.youtube.com/watch?v=o7BiGlUWomY

And...

https://www.youtube.com/watch?v=aYIwPu5oFic

***

How the hell did I get to that moment – stuck in an Asian nightclub, pondering life, and feeling overwhelmed?

It all started with the desire for freedom.

After graduating college with an Accounting major, I soon realized I didn't want to be an accountant. It was too boring, and I loved to create things. When I sat in a cubicle in the accounting office, I felt caged. "This couldn't be all there is to life," I thought.

I was hungry for more. Hungry for adventure. I didn't want to be another dude who just checked off boxes. You know the boxes I'm talking about. Go to college, get a job, buy a house, get married, have kids, buy a bigger house, get a promotion, retire, etc.

It all seemed so predictable...

So, I saved up just enough money to quit my job. I moved back home with my parents, but even then, I had just enough savings to last a few months.

I had to make something happen. "Now or never," I thought.

Scared and quickly running out of money, I did the only thing I could do: start learning.

I learned how to start a blog, and started one. Then, I learned copywriting, and tried to get clients.

The goal? Well, the long-term goal was to travel the world and achieve financial freedom. But my short-term goal was simply to make $2k a month. I knew if I could do that, I could move to Vietnam where there were tons of location-independent entrepreneurs.

(My friend had been living in Vietnam for a year, and raving about how he was learning so much about business and life from these entrepreneurs.)

I started off writing 500 word articles for $7.50 a pop. I remember calculating how many I needed to write per day to pay my rent. It was A LOT. And certainly not sustainable. But I kept learning and looking for better opportunities.

It took me about six months and a few lucky breaks. But once I started making $2k a month, I pulled the trigger and bought my plane ticket in May of 2014. I was set to leave at the end of July.

Scared, excited, and hopeful, I knew this could be a life-changing step on my journey.

But a week after I bought my ticket, I met Natalie. She was the first girl in years that I truly connected with. The problem? I knew I'd have to leave her…

***

You can also make the story more interesting by involving her and pausing at the right times.

So, how do you involve her? Ask her pointed questions throughout the story, so she feels like she's a part of it.
For example, "So I was at an improv show the other night – do you like improv? Well this was just about the funniest show I've been to. Maybe I'll take you to one some time! Anyway, I was at this show and…"

As for pausing? Well, you should never rush through your stories – especially the important parts. You see, people don't feel moved by your words – they feel moved by the spaces in between your words. Pausing for just a second or two here and there can be powerful.

***

"Guys, I'm gonna head home," I told the group. This first night in Asia had been a little more than I could handle.

I rushed out of the club and on to the street, in search of a taxi. The humidity and pollution flooded my senses once again. And that's when it hit me.

"What have I done?!" I thought. I'd flown all the way across the world to fulfill some dream of adventure, travel, and entrepreneurship. But maybe that's not what I wanted after all.

Maybe I should have stayed in Boston and made it work with Natalie. Maybe I should've gotten a real job, made normal friends, and lived a regular life.

But I couldn't turn back. Hell, I didn't even have enough money to fly back to the US.

I was on the other side of the globe, with only one person I knew in this huge city, and I had no choice but to keep going...

So I hopped in a Taxi, showed the driver a little sticky note with the address written in Vietnamese, and headed back to my friend's apartment. I wasn't sure if I had ruined my life or if I had finally gone too far.

I texted Natalie a sappy, "Wish I was back there hanging with you," and went to bed.

***

The way you tell a story is important, but you also need to do it in a way that attracts women.

Here are the components of a story that attracts her:

It Should Help You Connect With Her

The point of the story is to help you connect with the girl. So, your stories should be about you or something that happened to you. Otherwise, they won't do much in the way of connecting.

It Should Showcase Your Attractive Qualities

Remember the qualities we talked about in the last chapter?

(Dominance, sociability, altruism, adventurousness, appreciation of beauty, and sense of humor.)

These are the types of qualities you want to showcase in your stories. Don't worry about stuffing all of them in to every story. Aim to highlight 1-3.

It Should Be About Something She's Interested In

This is where baiting comes into play. If she asks you about a topic relevant to your story, tell it then –that's when it will have the most impact.

For example, if she asks you, "How did you end up moving to Vietnam?"

It Should End With a Bang

Try to end with the impact. Wrap everything up and have some type of takeaway.

***

"Hey bro, do you want to go to yoga?" My friend woke me up and asked if I wanted to head there with the guys. I had never tried yoga, and I was still feeling very overwhelmed – but I knew I needed some sort of "pick-me-up."

"Alright let's do it."

At yoga, I met a few more guys from the crew. This was an easier atmosphere to handle than the club. I felt a little more calm and relaxed.

Afterwards, we hit the local smoothie shop, "Juicy" to grab some smoothies.

I told the guys about my experience from the night before.

"Listen man," my friend began. "Being here, seeing all this, meeting these entrepreneurs – it's overwhelming at first. I was scared for my first few months."

"But this is just the beginning of everything. What you're going to learn is that the world is about to open up to you. No place is going to be off limits. And there are plenty of amazing women all around the globe."

As I talked to the guys, I began to feel a bit more comfortable. They had all been scared when they started traveling and getting into business. And they also had the similar goals of freedom, adventure, and financial success.
I could relate to these guys.
Right then, I decided: "You know what? I'm going to try to make this work. I'm going to give this a shot."

Those next few weeks were tough, as I got accustomed to Asia. I still missed Natalie, and I still wasn't sure if I made the right decision.

But as the days passed, Vietnam grew on me more and more. I realized, "This is the type of lifestyle and freedom I'd always wanted, so let me try and enjoy it."

Soon enough, I loved Vietnam and the people there. I started learning more, meeting amazing people, and having more success in business.

***

As I sit here writing this 2 years later from a beach in Playa Del Carmen, Mexico, I can say it for sure – it all turned out okay. More than okay. I've lived in 5 different countries since then, made amazing friends, and have no plans of stopping any time soon. Now, the world really is my oyster.

And if I'd retreated back home after that scary first night in Vietnam, I never would have made this amazing discovery.

And while it didn't work out with Natalie, I've met several amazing women from all around the world.

So I guess sometimes, you have to scare yourself a little bit. You have to destroy your life to let the next great thing happen.

And that's okay. Because you can build it back up better than you ever thought possible.

***

There's one more step to tell a story that hooks her in: You need to have a solid structure.

You see, every story has 4 basic elements. And if you've been following along to my story about Vietnam, you might have picked up on these elements.

Here are the 4 elements of a great story:

1) Introduction. You introduce the characters/environment in the story, and hook in your listener. For example, "The music bumped and the ground shook below me. I looked around in awe. I had just stepped into my first nightclub in Asia, after nearly 30 hours of travel. And I was scared."

2) Development. You share the characters' main struggles and obstacles. For example, "It took me about six months and a few lucky breaks. But once I started making $2k a month, I pulled the trigger and bought my plane ticket in May of 2014. I was set to leave at the end of July. But a week after I bought my ticket, I met Natalie. She was the first girl in years that I truly connected with. The problem? I knew I'd have to leave her…"

3) Climax. This is the turning point in the story. For example, "And that's when it hit me. 'Holy fuck. What have I done?!' I thought. I'd flown all the way across the world to fulfill some dream of adventure, travel, and entrepreneurship. But maybe that's not what I wanted after all."

4) Resolution. You wind the story down and wrap it up. It's the "come-down" from the climax. For example, "I decided to give Vietnam a real try, even though it was scary. So I guess sometimes, you have to scare yourself a little bit. You have to destroy your life to let the next great thing happen. And that's okay. Because you can build it back up better than you ever thought possible."

Let's recap how to tell a story that hooks her in:

1) Use the aspects of good storytelling (tell it as if you're living in, involve her, and use pauses)

2) Tell a story that attracts her (it should be about you and showcase your attractive qualities.

3) Nail the structure (introduction, development, climax, and resolution)

Action tip: Write a short story about something that has happened to you. Include the 4 elements of the story structure. Then, tell it aloud to yourself as if you were living it.

Part VI:
The Final Conversation

A Simple Habit to Improve Your Conversation Skills

"Are ya'll from America?"

My friend and I had just sat down at my favorite taco place in Medellin, Colombia – and we were ready to indulge...

That's when Walt – a 60 something year old guy from Kentucky (and the only other person in the restaurant) – approached us and started a conversation.

He seemed innocent enough at first. A fellow gringo just looking for some English-speaking conversation partners in a city where they're hard to come by.

But we soon realized this guy had no interest in talking to us – he only wanted to talk at us. After asking for our names, he went on a tangent about how his daughter dated a guy with the same name. This led to another tangent about how his daughter's boyfriend was an investor, and how he had actually invested a lot himself. Which led to a tangent about he had traveled the world. On and on he went.

All of this without our prompting. He went on for the entire length of our meal, with pretty much zero input from either of us. It was almost impressive the way he could ignore our clear signs of disinterest.

Now I'll ask you: Have you ever been guilty of this?

Maybe you don't go on for a half hour on random, self-absorbed tangents – but perhaps, from time to time, you focus a little too much on yourself and what you can gain, rather than truly engaging the other person and adding value to the conversation.

Or maybe you're so focused on saying the "right thing" and/or worrying about what the other person thinks of you, that you don't take the time to actually listen.

This is a big problem that a lot of guys face when talking to women.

Here's the thing: in order to connect with a woman, you need to remove the focus from yourself and put it on her. You need to be present and engaged in the conversation.

But in the process of trying to prove we're cool and worthy, we forget about this. We're inclined to keep dropping hints about how awesome and impressive we are.

All the while, the girl is thinking, "Wow this guy is full of himself."

The more you fall into these bad conversation habits, that harder it will be for you to connect with women.
So, how do you stop yourself from falling into these traps? How do you make it easier to connect with women?

There's one simple habit I give to a lot of my clients – and it works like a charm:

Try to learn 3 things about her.

In other words, you approach a girl with the intent to learn something new about her.

It could be any 3 things. But it's more powerful when the things aren't simple facts (like what she does, what her name is, etc.). Those are fine to start with, but you'll make a deeper connection if the things are based more on her emotions and the way she feels.

For example, here are a few things you could try to learn in a new conversation:

- Something she is passionate about

- Why she decided to live in a particular city

- What she likes (or dislikes) about her job

- A place she's traveled to – and how she felt about it

- What kind of music she's into

- What her aspirations are

- Something she's excited about

Think of a few yourself, and use some of these examples. In doing so, you'll build the habit – and start naturally engaging women in conversation, and improving your ability to connect with them.

You'll also avoid the trap of making the conversation all about you. You know, so you don't have to be like Walt from Kentucky.

Action Tip: For the next few days, focus on 3 things from everybody you talk to.

How to Genuinely Love Women

You've learned tons of conversation tactics throughout this book.

But, if you don't genuinely love women, none of it will matter.

In order to be truly successful with women you need to become a man who loves women.

You see, a woman can feel the difference when she's interacting with a man who genuinely loves women, and one who does not.

She quickly develops trust with the man who loves women. She can sense he has no ulterior motive, he enjoys the moment, he understands her, and he appreciates her beauty. And as a result, she is more comfortable moving things further with this man.

She never truly feels comfortable around the man who does not love women. She can sense he is not truly comfortable in her world, he is out for some ulterior motive (e.g. proving himself to himself or his friends), he doesn't understand her, and his mind is in another place. As a result, she usually doesn't want to move forward with this man.

And so, you need to learn how to love women.

Here's how things can change for you when you start genuinely loving women:

- You'll earn more trust, more quickly with women

- You'll have more enjoyment from your experiences

- Better relationships

- Warmer reactions and more flirtation

- Free yourself from bitterness towards women

- And a lot more...

But here's the thing: many guys find it difficult to genuinely love women. This is due to a few reasons:

Bitterness. They've been rejected or hurt in the past, and now they hold a grudge against women. They want to "get back" at women for all the pain they've caused.

Inexperience. They haven't dealt with women enough, and so they struggle to understand them. *Stubbornness.* They refuse to acknowledge that women are emotional creatures. They deal with problems and decisions differently they men do.

Stubborn men get bent out of shape when women don't act logically.

Insecurity. They're pursuing women to "complete" themselves or make themselves feel like they're "okay".

If you want to love women, you need to work through these things. You see, any man can love women when he's having tons of sex, getting eye contact left and right, and hanging with high quality girls. But you also need to learn to love them in the tough times.

So, let's talk about how you can genuinely love women...

Accept Responsibility

We talked about this at the beginning, in the chapter on "Taking Responsibility for Your Life" (so go back, check it out, and do the action step if you need a reminder).

This is key for loving women. You must not blame them for your failures, nor allow yourself to become bitter if things don't go your way.

Understand that Women Are Emotional

Women are emotional creatures, and you can't blame them for it. The way you analyze situations and problems is much different – much more logical – than the way women do.

And so, you must cater to their emotions when interacting with and attracting them. Remember: women care more about the way you make them feel than your "stats" and accomplishments. That is the secret to connecting. When they feel that you understand this, they'll relate to you more and mentally put you in the group of guys who "get it".

You also need to be aware of this in your general interactions with women. She might say one thing one day based on how she feels, then say something completely different the next day – just because her emotions shifted. You need to have patience here.

Appreciate Her Beauty

When you're interacting with a beautiful woman, a lot of things can be going through your head...

"Does she like me?" "Should I try to kiss her?" "What should I talk about?" "What if she thinks I'm boring?"

All of these thoughts rob you of being in the moment – and she can sense it. Instead of focusing on these thoughts, focus on appreciating her beauty.

What do you like about her? Do her eyes draw you in and captivate you? Is her smile contagious? Is her rhythm sexy? Does she make you laugh? Bring these thoughts to the forefront of your mind.

As you appreciate her inner and outer beauty, you'll be more in tune with your natural male instincts.

For me, it always brings a smile to my face and leads me to make strong eye contact. It allows me to be more free-flowing and in the moment as well.

Have a Mission Outside of Women

You need to have a mission in life outside of women. Otherwise, you will be too tempted to give up on your passions and your direction in life and focus completely on women. Women will sense that they are the center of your world, and you won't be able to genuinely love them. Instead, you will rely on them to fill needs that they cannot fill. You will mistake your neediness for love, and this will undermine your relationships.

Loving women is a tough concept to grasp. If you don't have a lot of experience or you hold bitterness, it's even tougher. But this is something you must put into practice. The more you come to love women, the better and more fulfilling your dating life, conversations, and relationships will be.

The Final Talk

Hey man, you've made it. We're almost at the end...

But let me ask you this: Have you taken the action steps at the end of the chapters? Have you started putting this newfound knowledge to work in your life?

If you do, I can promise you'll see big changes. You'll improve your ability to communicate, talk, and flirt with women. And you'll see some satisfying results in your dating and sex life, as well as your ability to network with other people.

But if you don't, you'll be right back to where you started when you picked up this book.

I trust that if you've read this far, you'll make the right decision.

What you'll discover is that people are interesting, life is exciting, and the only limits that exist are those you put on yourself.

The conversation tools in this book have helped me travel the world, start a business, connect with amazing people, and meet beautiful women from more countries than I can count. It's been quite the journey.

I hope that for you, these conversation tools can help you achieve your deepest desires. More than just with women – but also in every area of your life.

So, use them wisely, take some massive action, and crush it.

Bonus Chapter: 20 Questions to Ask a Girl on the First Date

We've all had awkward first dates.

Sometimes, it feels like you just can't break through and connect with the girl. You're stuck in small talk and can't get out. B

ut there ARE ways you can "escape" small talk and start connecting. A big part of that is asking the right questions.

So, here are 20 questions to put in your back pocket the next time you have a first date.

These questions will help you open up the conversation, learn about her, and give you a chance to listen and relate back.

(Note: Don't try to stuff all of these questions into your first dates. Choose a few of them that you like and weave them into the conversation to make things more interesting when things die down.

1) What are you passionate about?

2) What do you find sexiest in a guy?

3) What's your dream job?

4) What's one thing I wouldn't guess about you?

5) If you could wake up anywhere in the world tomorrow, where would it be?

6) What kind of things make you laugh the hardest?

7) What was your last big adventure?

8) What's something you've always wanted to do?

9) What do you absolutely love to do?

10) Would you consider yourself a sexual person?

11) Have you ever had sex in a public place?

12) What's your favorite place you've traveled to?

13) If your apartment were on fire, what 2 things would you save?

14) What kind of music do you listen to?

15) If you could go back to what time period in history, what would it be?

16) Do you cook? What's your favorite meal?

17) What brought you to this city?

18) How did you get into what you're doing now?

19) What's your favorite movie of all time?

20) What's your favorite book of all time?

Your Next Step

If you apply what you learn in this book, you can go out there and have a great dating life.

But some of you may want more help and even to fast-track your success. After all, going at it alone isn't easy, even if you have the right tools and knowledge.

That's why I've teamed up with my good friend, How to Beast, to create the Beastly Lifestyle Mentorship program.

It's a group coaching program where we personally mentor you, answer your questions, hold you accountable, and help accelerate your road to a great dating life and legendary lifestyle. We've been running it for nearly a year, and guys have gotten great results from it.

If that sounds like something you're interested in, just navigate to the application here:

https://bit.ly/Lifestyle_application

If you seem like a good fit, we'll email you to schedule a call and give you more details.

I look forward to chatting with you and helping you further accelerate your dating goals!

About the Author

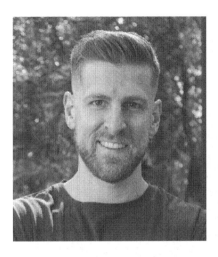

Dave Perrotta is a bestselling author, entrepreneur, and YouTuber—on his channel, he shows men how to get the girls they want and achieve a high-value lifestyle.

His other bestselling books include:

The Lifestyle Blueprint: How to Talk to Women, Build Your Social Circle, and Grow Your Wealth.

Struggling to create a lifestyle of great friends, beautiful women, and financial freedom? This book lays out the blueprint to do all of these things and live a lifestyle you love. It will drastically change your outlook on the world, spike your motivation, and help you reach the potential you didn't even know you had.

The Hook Up Handbook: 28 Fundamentals to Keep Her Coming Back for More

Struggling to close the deal with girls and give them the types of hookups they crave? Want to be able to blow them out of the water with every hookup and have them saying you're the "best they've ever had"? This book is your answer.

How to Reach Me

If you've got a question about the book or how to apply any of the concepts, the best way to reach me is either through an Instagram DM or an email.

- Instagram: **www.instagram.com/dave.perrotta/**
- Email: **Dave@postgradcasanova.com**

I love chatting with readers, so feel free to reach out, and I'll get back to you as soon as I can!

If you'd like to see more of my content on video, check it out here:

www.youtube.com/daveperrotta

You can also check out my TikTok, where I post daily videos and dating skits:

TikTok: @daveperrotta

I post new videos here every single week to help you level up your lifestyle and dating life.

A Parting Gift

There's no doubt in my mind that you're well on your way to mastering and flirting like a Casanova!

But in order to take the next step with a girl, you need to know how to text her the right way.

That's why I created the **Texting "Cheat Sheet"**. It contains 18 powerful texts to capture her attention, get her on a date, and turn her on.

Inside you will learn:

- 3 proven texts for setting up the date

- 3 texts that turn her on and make her think about you

- A proven text that gets her to respond every time (even if she's been ignoring you)

- Simple online dating text openers for Tinder, OkCupid, etc.

Download it here:
postgradcasanova.com/conversation-casanova-free-ebook/

Bonus Epilogue

I write this to you from my home office in Mexico City. It's February of 2021, and it's been nearly five years since I wrote this book.

A lot has changed in that time—and this book has become more successful than I ever could've imagined.

Between the paperback, audiobook, and Kindle, it's sold over 50,000 copies, and continues to sell well to this day.

In the process, it's helped tens of thousands of men to improve their conversations, flirt with girls, and start becoming the men they've always known they could be.

My hope is that you do the same.

Improving with women is a journey, and one that has completely changed my life. It's made me reconsider what is possible, and stretch beyond my original self-imposed limitations.

It's a journey, unfortunately, that many men either give up early on, or never even truly start in the first place. They settle with women they aren't all that crazy about, and it leads to weak relationships that go nowhere.

Don't be one of these men. Seek the best out of life, and don't settle just because it's the path of least resistance.

Implementing what you learn in this book won't be easy—but it will be worth it.

So, go forward, live dangerously, and enjoy the ride. Life is so much more fun when you have faith in yourself than when you live scared.

Made in the USA
Las Vegas, NV
23 October 2022